BDJ Clinician's Guides

This series enables clinicians at all stages of their careers to remain well informed and up to date on key topics across all fields of clinical dentistry. Each volume is superbly illustrated and provides concise, highly practical guidance and solutions. The authors are recognised experts in the subjects that they address. The *BDJ Clinician's Guides* are trusted companions, designed to meet the needs of a wide readership. Like the *British Dental Journal* itself, they offer support for undergraduates and newly qualified, while serving as refreshers for more experienced clinicians. In addition they are valued as excellent learning aids for postgraduate students.

The BDJ Clinicians' Guides are produced in collaboration with the British Dental Association, the UK's trade union and professional association for dentists.

Stephen Davies • Emma Beecroft
Justin Durham
Editors

Temporomandibular Disorders in Primary Dental Care

The Clinical Guide

Springer

Editors
Stephen Davies
Division of Dentistry
University of Manchester
Manchester, UK

Emma Beecroft
School of Dental Sciences
Newcastle University
Newcastle upon Tyne, UK

Justin Durham
School of Dental Sciences
Newcastle University
Newcastle upon Tyne, UK

ISSN 2523-3327 ISSN 2523-3335 (electronic)
BDJ Clinician's Guides
ISBN 978-3-032-01300-2 ISBN 978-3-032-01301-9 (eBook)
https://doi.org/10.1007/978-3-032-01301-9

This Springer imprint is published by the registered company Springer Nature Switzerland AG
The registered company address is: Gewerbestrasse 11, 6330 Cham, Switzerland

Preface

In 1993, at the invitation of the British Dental Association (BDA), Robin Gray, Alan Quayle and I wrote a book on Temporomandibular Disorders (TMD). This was published in 1995 as the first book in their clinical guide series. This second edition acts as a contemporary guide reflecting the development of understanding which has taken place over the 30 years since our original publication.

Our brief in 1993 was to demystify and make TMD accessible to dentists working in primary care. It proved to be a successful publication, leading to a second print run and being translated into German. Whether it encouraged dentists to diagnose and care for this group of patients is much less certain.

We were aware, at the time of writing, that care for patients living with a temporomandibular disorder needed to move away from the 'identify *the cause* to affect *a cure*' model.

In the original Chapter 11, we wrote:

'treatment must be appropriate to the patient as a person'
'there is no single panacea'
'the threshold concept is important'
'what we may achieve is a reduction of symptoms to a point at which they cease to concern the patient'

We knew 30 years ago that there was much we didn't yet know. But, even then, we realised and recognised that effective and empathetic management had to be patient centred. Classification of temporomandibular disorders had also begun to move away from considering this group of conditions as a single disorder.

I am lucky and privileged to been able to observe the progress that has been made over the last three decades. This progress is partly due to a better general understanding of the pathophysiology and biopsychosocial nature of chronic or persistent pain, and partly due to specific work into the diagnostic criteria and management of TMD.

It is the hope of the editors and contributors of this book that the clearer guidance that we have been able to bring to this second edition will empower dental clinicians to help this large and important group of patients.

Manchester, UK
2023

Stephen Davies

Contents

Introduction

Stephen Davies

1 Why Should Dental Clinicians Be Interested in Temporomandibular Disorders?

All dental clinicians have patients who are suffering from temporomandibular disorders [TMD]; the prevalence of TMD [1] in the general population makes this inevitable.

However, not all of these patients will have their condition diagnosed and then appropriately managed.

The first aim of this book is to empower dental clinicians to be able to recognise and diagnose TMD.

The advantages of this ability are:

1. To be able to provide or organise help for the patient suffering from TMD
2. To avoid mis-diagnosis, based upon a clinician's current level of knowledge [Diagnostic Bias]
3. To be able to consider a pause of restorative treatment, at an appropriate juncture, if the patient develops a TMD

This book hopes to illustrate how TMD can significantly affect a patient's quality of life. These are a group of patients who will justifiably look to the dental profession for help.

Diagnostic Bias is a recognisable problem in the medical profession [2]; one can only diagnose within one's knowledge base. It is the view of the authors that an inability to diagnose TMD can lead to a clinician providing inappropriate and often irreversible, invasive treatments. The motive of a caring dental clinician will be to try to help the patient, but even well-meaning and good quality treatment for the

S. Davies (✉)
Division of Dentistry, University of Manchester, Manchester, UK
e-mail: stephen.j.davies@manchester.ac.uk

S. Davies et al. (eds.), *Temporomandibular Disorders in Primary Dental Care*,
BDJ Clinician's Guides, https://doi.org/10.1007/978-3-032-01301-9_1

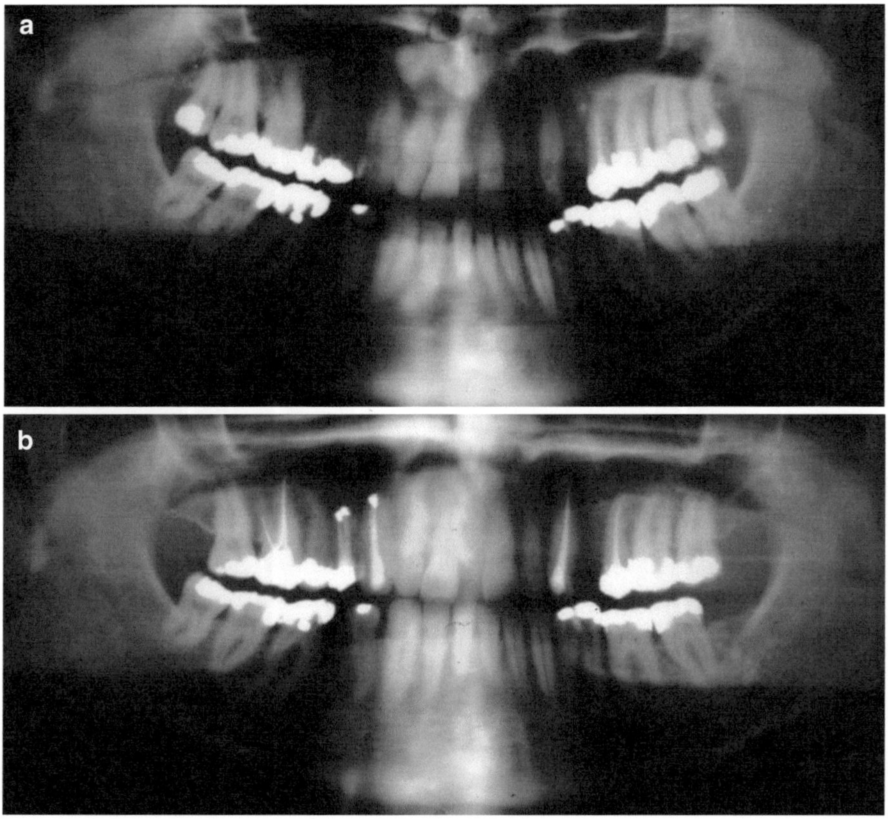

Fig. 1 (**a**) Pre-operative radiograph. (**b**) Post-operative radiograph demonstrating multiple dental treatments unsuccessfully trialled to manage pain eventually diagnosed as TMD: Dental extractions 3, root canal treatments 5, apicectomies 2 and crowns 3

wrong diagnosis is mistreatment. Potentially every TMD clinic will frequently see patients who have had endodontic treatment and extractions in a misguided attempt to reduce the symptoms of TMD (Fig. 1).

If a patient develops the signs and symptoms of TMD during restorative or orthodontic treatment, then it will help the clinicians and the patient if this is recognised immediately. The symptoms can then be addressed, often by simple measures covered in the "Management" chapter, including reassurance, explanation and a treatment break. If TMD develops during restorative treatment, it may not be the *product* of that treatment [for instance, a new occlusal scheme], it may be the *process* of the treatment [i.e. maintaining a wide mouth opening whilst a bridge is being prepared]. So symptomatic conservative TMD management should be the first response, rather than altering the occlusion of the new restorations.

2 What Are Temporomandibular Disorders?

TMD is a generic term covering a range of conditions. TMD does not stand for temporomandibular joint dysfunction; many TMD patients have healthy, comfortable and functioning temporomandibular joints [TMJs].

The differential diagnoses within TMD have distinct diagnostic criteria, which will be outlined in Chapter "Examination and Diagnosis for Temporomandibular Disorder". It is possible for patients to present with multiple TMD diagnoses, and it will be seen through this book that not all TMD need an intervention.

TMD is an abbreviation of temporomandibular disorders. It is important that dentists do not consider TMD a single condition. As will be seen as the reader progresses through the chapters of this book, there are marked differences between TMD sub-diagnoses, e.g. myofascial pain or a disc displacement without reduction, although, maybe confusingly, both of these diagnoses may be associated with pain and restricted opening. These different diagnoses will mean the tissues that are affected will not be the same; the presenting signs and symptoms will be different, and consequently, appropriate management will be different.

Notes on Terminology

Within this text, if an author does refer to TMD in the singular, it will always be followed by a relevant sub-diagnosis.

For the purpose of the book, TMD will stand for temporomandibular disorders.

From a pain perspective, "persistent" and "chronic" both mean pain which lasts for 3 months or more. This book will use the accepted clinical terminology of persistent pain. It is important, however, that clinicians understand that patients may be more comfortable, understand more clearly and refer to the term "chronic" pain. Several definitions of TMD exist, but they can be paraphrased as a "*collective term embracing a number of clinical problems that involve the masticatory muscles, the TMJ and associated structures*" [3, 4].

The terms "the masticatory muscles, the TMJs and associated structures" could be taken to be a description of the articulatory system, which is the third component of the stomatognathic or masticatory system (Fig. 2).

The first two elements of the masticatory system, the teeth and periodontal system (periodontium), are universally well taught in dental under-graduate programs.

The articulatory system is not always covered to the same depth, so, it is not uncommon for a newly qualified dentist to be unsure of the functional anatomy of the TMJs, the function of the muscles of mastication or the subject of occlusion (Fig. 3).

A good place to start understanding the function of each component of the articulatory system is to consider what an engineer would call each element. In using this analogy, the authors are not suggesting that the articulatory system should ever be considered to be a machine. ["A machine is a system that is not the result of a fertilised egg"] [5]. Unlike a machine, living systems [our patients] demonstrate adaptive capability. Because of this ability, the reader of Chapter "Management" on

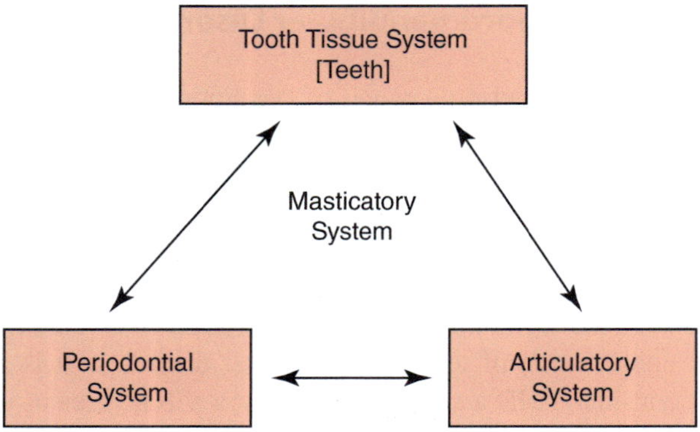

Fig. 2 The components of the stomatognathic or masticatory system

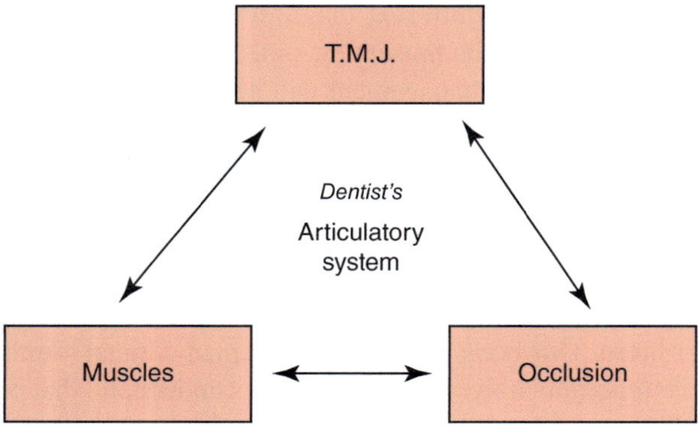

Fig. 3 The components of the articulatory system

management will see that part of the strategy is to try to improve the patient's adaptive capability (Fig. 4).

So, one way of considering TMD is to see them as a:

- Discomfort in
- Dysfunction of
- …….the articulatory system.

It, therefore, will be no surprise to the reader that there is chapter on the examination of the articulatory system in this book, this can be considered as a screening protocol for TMD. Although our protocol and similar ones are used in secondary care referral centres, it is equally applicable to primary care. The use of such protocols is important as early diagnosis, that can be made in primary care, will benefit the patient. There is a worldwide consensus that the majority of TMD patients should be diagnosed within primary care, and considerable efforts are being made to provide a quick and simple diagnostic criteria for general dental practitioners [GDPs] to use [6].

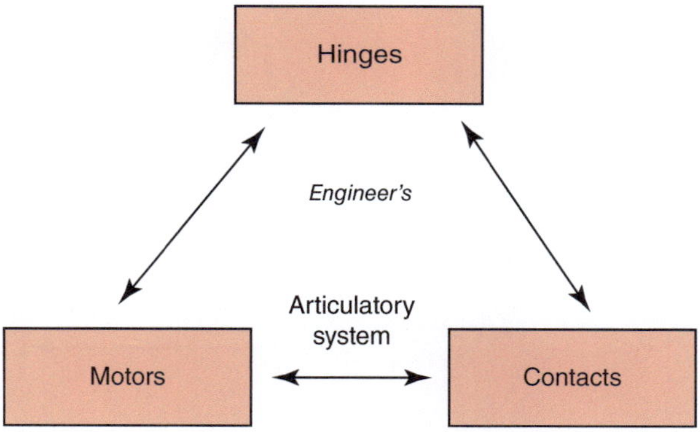

Fig. 4 The engineer's interpretation of the articulatory system

One of the aims of this book is provide general dental practitioners (GDPs) with quick and easy examination protocol in order to both screen their patients for TMD (Chapter "Examination and Diagnosis of Temporomandibular Disorders") and to help them make a diagnosis for their patients with the signs and symptoms of TMD.

This early intervention is especially important for patients suffering from TMD sub-diagnosis myofascial pain, which is essentially a myalgia. The reason for this is that the longer a patient is left suffering from this condition, the more likely that they are to develop the complications associated with persistency, in particular central sensitisation. Persistency is associated with pain, loss of sleep, anxiety, depression and increased muscle tension, all of which will have a negative effect on the experience for the patient (Chapter "Examination and Diagnosis of Temporomandibular Disorders") (Fig. 5).

Chapter "Functional Anatomy and Pain Science" of this book covers functional anatomy and pain science focussing on trigeminal pain pathways. An understanding of how nociceptive (pain) messages are processed and transmitted by the body and how persistent or chronic pain can result is essential to enable clinicians to help those living with pain. Dental clinicians are more used to diagnosing the causes of acute pain, exposure to managing persistent pain issues is less common. The ability to make an early diagnosis of TMD has been shown to be a significant predictor of a good prognosis (Chapter "Examination and Diagnosis of Temporomandibular Disorders") [7]. It is no surprise that persistent pain that is experienced in the head/face can have a profound effect upon the wellbeing of a patient; after all the head is the only part of the body that contains all five senses, and it is central to consciousness and being *ourself.*

As a postscript to this introduction to persistent pain, it should be remembered that not all TMD are painful.

The art and science of dentistry is much more than repairing, replacing and moving teeth, together with looking after the periodontal structures. As oral physicians, as well as surgeons, we need an understanding of both the articulatory and pain

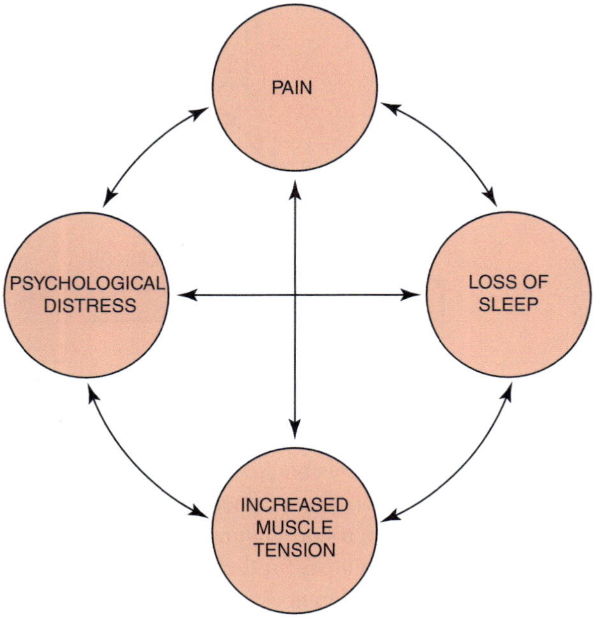

Fig. 5 Some of the multidirectional problems affecting the patient with persistent pain

systems and the ills that can affect them. The authors of this book hope that this book will contribute to that understanding.

This clinical guide examines TMD under the following headings:

3 Functional Anatomy, Pain Science and Pathways and Classification

This will provide an understanding of the functional anatomy and how crucial it is to a clinician's competence. In addition, the complex subject of "pain" will be explained, from the mechanism of nociception through to the subjective experience of pain that is felt by the brain. There are, also, descriptions of the function and effects of persistent pain.

4 Examination of the Articulatory System

As stated, the ability to be able to examine the elements of the articulatory system is crucial to a clinician's ability to make an accurate diagnosis. This chapter provides a quick and easy examination protocol that can be adopted by dental clinicians.

5 Psychosocial Considerations

Pain is a complex experience, this chapter will help the reader understand the phenomenon of chronic or persistent pain. This is essential to enable a dental clinician to support and help *those with persistent pain issues related to their* TMD. Although this represents a greater clinical challenge than removing a necrotic pulp for a patient suffering the *acute pain* of pulpitis, it is a very valuable service that our caring profession can make.

6 Management

As the reader will expect, having described the anatomy, signs and symptoms and differential diagnoses of TMD, this chapter explores the different therapies available to manage these multifactorial conditions. The fact that supported self-management will feature may surprise the reader, which it shouldn't when we consider how our profession treats periodontal disease.

7 Surgical Interventions in Temporomandibular Disorders

This chapter looks at how our oral and maxillofacial surgical colleagues can help the small number of TMD patients who need a surgical intervention. It has two aims: firstly, to inform the GDP the range of surgical interventions, from the minimally invasive, through open surgeries including TMJ joint replacement; secondly, the detail given will provide an invaluable resource to those undertaking an oral and maxillofacial surgery speciality training program.

8 Case Histories

Different treatment modalities are presented through case histories, covering a wide range of TMD patients.

9 The Role of the GDP in TMD

This book is written mainly for GDPs, and this chapter is written by a dentist who has devoted the majority of his time working in a general dental practice. The role of the GDP in the management of TMD is very important, and it is hoped that this book will empower and encourage GDPs to fulfil this role. As a specialist in restorative dentistry [8], he is also able to discuss occlusion and TMD, hopefully casting some light on this often confusing and contentious subject.

References

1. Valesan, et al. Prevalence of temporomandibular joint disorders: a systematic review and meta-analysis. Clin Oral Investig. 2021;25:441–53. https://doi.org/10.1007/s00784-020-03710-w.
2. Cain DM, Detsky AS. Everyone's a little bit biased (even physicians). JAMA. 2008;299(24):2893–5.
3. De Leeuw R, editor. Orofacial pain; guidelines for assessment, diagnosis, and management. 4th ed. Chicago: Quintessence Pub. Co.; 2008. p. 129–204.
4. Greene CS. Managing the care of patients with TMD: new guidelines for care. J Am Dent Assoc. 2010;141:1086–8.
5. "The private life of the brain: emotions, consciousness, and the secret of Self" Prof Susan Greenfield.
6. Durham, et al. Constructing the brief diagnostic criteria for temporomandibular disorders (bDC/TMD) for field testing. J Oral Rehabil. 2024;51(5):785–94. https://doi.org/10.1111/joor.13652. Epub 2023 Dec 27.
7. Durham J, et al. Temporomandibular disorder patients' journey through care. Community Dent Oral Epidemiol. 2011;39:532–41.
8. Davies S. A guide to good occlusal practice. Springer Nature; 2022. s

Functional Anatomy and Pain Science

David Edwards, Joanna Matthan, James Allison,
Emma Beecroft, Chris Penlington, and Justin Durham

1 Introduction

An understanding of the structural and functional anatomy of the temporomandibular complex is crucial for developing clinical acumen. The anatomy of the region can appear complex, and considering the fact that pain can both radiate and refer to other regions, clinicians need to have an understanding of the anatomy and its topography to be able to interpret and interrogate clinical presentations of pain. Overlapping or mimicking clinical conditions may result in failure to diagnose temporomandibular disorders (TMD) or misdiagnosing a mimicking pathology as a TMD, both of which result in poor outcomes for patients. For this reason, structure and function relating to the preauricular region (also known as the temporomandibular region) cannot be isolated from each other. Understanding the function of this region and possible pathology requires a sound underpinning knowledge of structural anatomy and pathophysiology; this is explored in this section.

The original version of the chapter has been revised. A correction to this chapter can be found at https://doi.org/10.1007/978-3-032-01301-9_9

D. Edwards (✉) · J. Allison · E. Beecroft · C. Penlington · J. Durham
School of Dental Sciences, Newcastle University, Newcastle upon Tyne, UK
e-mail: david.edwards@newcastle.ac.uk; james.allison@newcastle.ac.uk; emma.beecroft@newcastle.ac.uk; chris.penlington@newcastle.ac.uk; justin.durham@newcastle.ac.uk

J. Matthan
Newcastle University Medicine Malaysia (NUMed), Johor, Malaysia
e-mail: joanna.matthan2@newcastle.edu.my

S. Davies et al. (eds.), *Temporomandibular Disorders in Primary Dental Care*, BDJ Clinician's Guides, https://doi.org/10.1007/978-3-032-01301-9_2

2 Overview of the Temporomandibular Joint and Associated Structures

The temporomandibular joint (TMJ; Fig. 1a–c) is a bilateral diarthrodial synovial joint or *ginglymoarthrodial* joint and is formed at the mandibular (or glenoid) fossa of the temporal bone and the condyle (head) of the mandible. As a

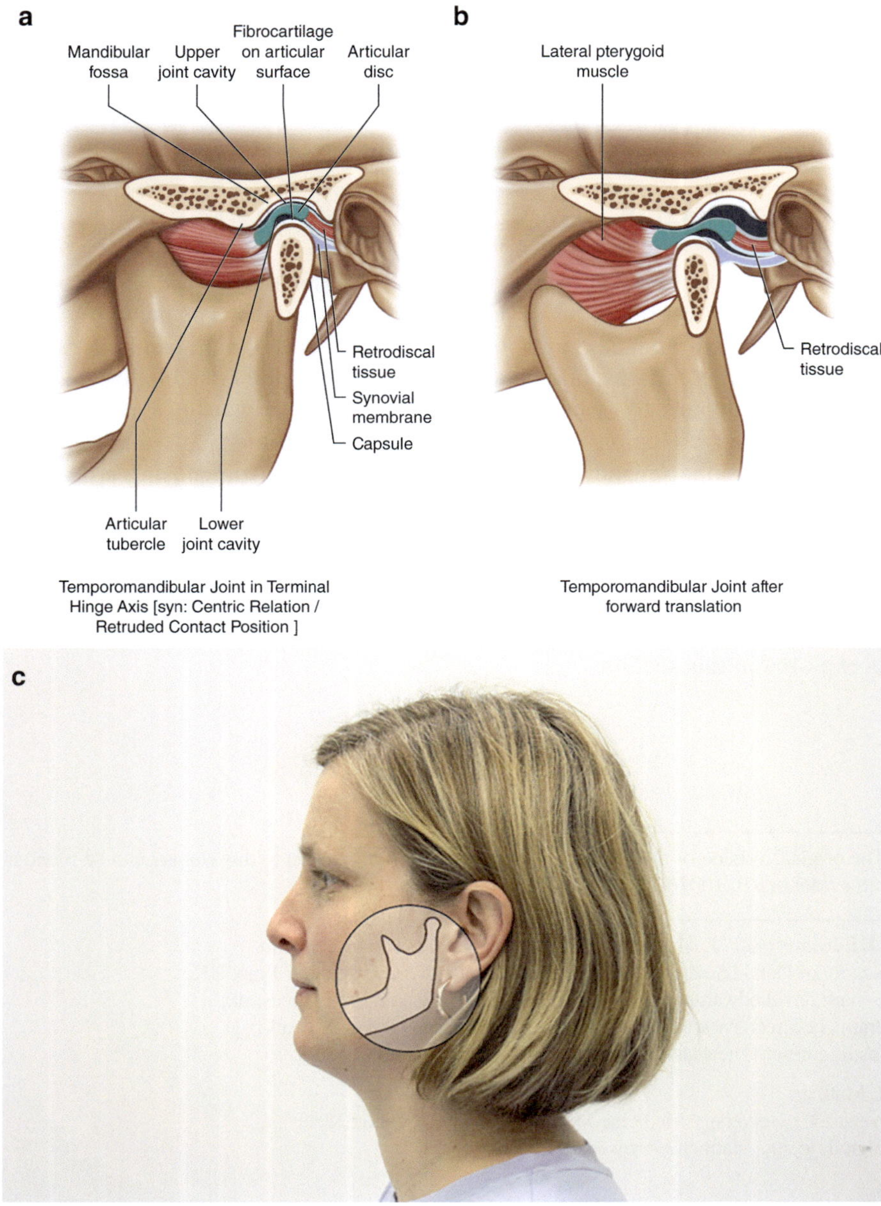

Fig. 1 Temporomandibular joint and articular disk

composite anatomical joint, one element of it is a hinge (i.e. *ginglymus or axial*) and the other a simple sliding (i.e. *arthrodial*) motion, shown as blue arrows in Fig. 1b. The gliding and hinge functions are enhanced by the insertion of a fibro-cartilaginous articular disc between the mandibular condyle and the mandibular fossa of the temporal bone. The interlinked movements possible at this joint occur within a cavity divided into two by the articular disc. This is a relatively complex structure which creates an upper (superior) and lower (inferior) joint space. The articular surfaces of both joint spaces are covered with fibrous tissue, and the joint capsule attaches to the margins of the articular surface, with accessory ligaments further stabilising the joint.

Despite being primarily a hinge joint, a gliding movement (or translation) also occurs at the TMJ. Movements at the joint are primarily produced by the supramandibular muscles, via attachments to the skull, which are mainly elevators of the mandible. The inframandibular muscles lower the mandible. The high masticatory forces produced by these muscles are dissipated, due to the shape of the articular structures, mainly through the teeth to the bones of the face and skull base.

3 The Temporomandibular Joint Complex

The bilateral TMJs are the only freely movable joints of the skull and are synovial. There are several features of the TMJ that must be understood to fully appreciate their structure and function: (1) osteology and articular surfaces, (2) fibrous capsule and intrinsic ligaments, (3) articular disc, (4) extrinsic ligaments, (5) movements at the joint, (6) muscles that move the joint, (7) jaw opening and closing cycle, (8) neurovascular supply and (9) functions of the joint. Each of these will be looked at briefly in turn.

1. *Osteology and Articular Surfaces*

The bilateral temporomandibular joints (TMJ) are comprised of the mandibular fossa (aka the glenoid fossa or the articular fossa) above and the head of the mandible (or mandibular condyle) below. The TMJ is diarthrodial synovial and paired, i.e. one part cannot move without the other. The articular surfaces of the joint are between the head of the mandible and the mandibular fossa on the articular part of the squamous part of the temporal bone.

The mandibular fossa is a depression on the temporal bone. Oval in shape, its anteroposterior dimension is lesser than its mediolateral dimension, and thus the latter is more relevant. The articular surface is limited anteriorly on the squamous temporal bone by the articular eminence. The articular eminence (or tubercle) on the zygomatic arch is a transversely elliptical prominence, curved in the sagittal plane and tilted forwards towards the occlusal plane at a 25-degree angle. It forms most of the articular surface of the mandibular fossa and varies in steepness, becoming flatter in the edentulous. On its posterior aspect, the fossa extends medially as far as the squamotympanic fissure and laterally the postglenoid tubercle, as the posterior part of the mandibular fossa is non-articular. The tympanic plate is the posterior limit. On its medial aspect, the glenoid plane forms a shallow ridge. It is worth noting that the fossa is not the same shape as the condyle.

The mandibular head is convex in shape and elliptical (and highly variable in size and angulation, with intraindividual differences also possible); it is constricted below at the condylar neck. The pterygoid fovea is anterior to this on the neck of the mandible. The articular surface is slightly curved and tilts forwards to the occlusal plane at a 25-degree angle and extends primarily around the anterior and superior rims of the head. The posterior surface is non-articular and, on occasion, separated from the articular surface by a ridge.

The narrow mandibular neck joins the mandibular knuckle-shaped head (or condyle) to the mandibular ramus. The pterygoid fovea is on anterior surface of the neck. It is noteworthy that there is considerable variation in both size and angulation between individuals and additionally between the right and left sides. Fibrocartilage covers the articular surfaces, not hyaline cartilage.

The jaw joint can be considered a weight-bearing joint, based on Newtonian mechanics. For instance, the left condyle must be able to support a load of over 300 N with a vertical bite force of 500 N on the first right molar. The non-working mandibular head is more loaded that that on the working side.

2. *Fibrous Capsule and Intrinsic Ligaments*

The capsule is tough and fibrous and completely surrounds the articular disc (aka meniscus). Tight fibres originating from the lower part of the TMJ attach the mandibular head to the disc. Looser fibres on the upper aspect of the joint attach the disc to the temporal bone. Consequently, as the disc attaches independently to both the temporal bone and the mandibular head, the capsule in effect resembles two capsules. Attached superiorly to the squamotympanic fissure and squamous bone around the margin of upper articular surface, the capsule extends from the articular tubercle to the squamotympanic fissure and between the medial glenoid eminence and lateral margin of articular eminence back to post glenoid process. Posteriorly, it is associated with the bilaminar zone of the articular disc, the retrodiscal zone. Inferior to this, it is attached just below the articular surface.

The capsule is lined with synovial membrane in all non-articular areas responsible for secreting the synovial fluid. It does not extend to cover the disc or other articular surfaces.

The capsule is strengthened by an intrinsic ligament called the lateral temporomandibular ligament. This is a thick band of fibrous tissue that extends from the lateral pole of the articular tubercle on the root of the zygomatic process of the temporal bone to the lateral and posterior border of the mandibular neck at an angle of 45-degrees. The ligament is thought to prevent posterior displacement of the mandibular head at rest. It does not appear to be well developed in the edentulous.

3. *Articular Disc*

An articular disc separates the two surfaces and divides the joint cavity into an upper and lower compartment. This disc is a plate of dense fibrocartilage (fibrous connective tissue) dividing the joint completely, and the shape is thought to centre the disc on the mandibular head (or condyle). A thick margin surrounding it forms a peripheral annulus. Its central depression on the lower surface accommodates the mandibular head. The disc blends with the capsule of the joint laterally and medially. On its anterior aspect, it is attached to the squamous temporal bone and the capsule. It divides into two laminae on the posterior aspect. The disc has in the past been described as bearing likeness to a schoolboy's peaked cap. Essentially, this translates to the upper surface of the disc being concavo-convex or saddle-shaped in an anterior-to-posterior direction and the inferior surface being concave to accommodate for the shape of the mandibular condyle. Its thickness is not uniform. However, the four zones of the articular disc, each a band of variable thickness, are consistent, with the thickest and widest being the posterior band. An anterior thickening is separated by a thin intermediate zone (the thinnest zone), and there is further thicker zone on the anterior aspect anterior. The arrangement where a thin intermediate zone is positioned between two thicker ones allows the disc some flexibility and for it to change its shape from concave to convex whilst moving forwards.

4. *Extrinsic Ligaments*

The ligaments associated with the TMJ help manage the forces associated with it and facilitate proprioceptive functions. There are two extrinsic ligaments: (1) the *sphenomandibular ligament*, a thin and flat band descending from the spine of the sphenoid and widening at its insertion on the lingula of the mandibular foramen, is likely to be the more significant of the two, and (2) the *stylomandibular ligament,* a thickened band of deep cervical fascia, attaches between the styloid process and the angle of the mandible and may be the less important of the two as its position and orientation do not allow it to mechanically limit normal movements of the mandible. The sphenomandibular ligament, on the other hand, is taut when the jaw is half open but has a ca 5 mm slack in the ligament when the jaw is closed. It also has important relations, with the chorda tympani lying medial to it at its upper end, the medial pterygoid lying inferomedial to it and the lateral pterygoid and auriculotemporal nerves laterally to it. Further, it is separated from the mandibular neck inferior to the lateral pterygoid by the maxillary artery; the inferior alveolar nerves and vessels as well as the parotid separate it from the ramus of the mandible. These neurovascular structures pierce the ligament at this point. A final important relation of the sphenomandibular ligament is that it is separated from the pharynx by a pharyngeal vein and fat.

5. *Movements at the Joint*

There are two types of movement possible at any joint separated by a disc (which is the primary function of the disc): hinge and rotation (aka translation). The hinge movement occurs in the inferior joint compartment. Here, only the head of the mandible moves, and the disc remains stationary and in contact with the squamous temporal bone. Translation occurs in the upper, superior joint compartment, where the mandibular head and the disc move forwards synchronously in a manner where the disc is in constant contact with the mandibular head—the movement of both are relative to the squamous temporal bone. These two movements occur concurrently in a cycle of mandibular depression and elevation, and only very rarely occur simultaneously.

6. *Muscles That Move the Joint*

The muscles that move the jaw fall into two broad categories: those that elevate the mandible (aka muscles of mastication or the supramandibular muscles) and those that depress the mandible (aka the inframandibular muscles). Movement of the jaw can only occur through attachments on the cranium or the hyoid bone. As moving the jaw, the masticatory muscles are relevant in cranial fractures as the strong pull of these muscles, usually resisted when the cranial bones are attached between, may result in bony displacements if a fracture occurs between the attachment sites of a muscle or muscles.

There are four supramandibular muscles (or muscles of mastication) shown in Fig. 2. These are the (1) *masseter* (Fig. 2a), a multipennate elevator of the jaw, which is attached between the external surface of the ramus of the mandible and the zygomatic arch; (2) *temporalis* (Fig. 2b), a bipennate elevator and retractor of the jaw, which is attached between the coronoid process and retromolar fossa to the temporal fossa between the temporal lines; (3) *medial pterygoid* (Fig. 2c), a jaw elevator attached between the internal surface of the ramus of the mandible and the medial surface of the medial pterygoid plate; and (4) *lateral pterygoid* (Fig. 2c), primarily a jaw depressor but also an elevator, which is attached between the anterior surface of the condylar process of the mandible and the base of skull, greater wing of sphenoid and lateral surface of the pterygoid. The lateral pterygoid has two parts to it: the lower part of the muscle is a jaw depressor, indirectly via protraction. The upper part of the muscle elevates.

There are four inframandibular muscles. These are the (1) *digastric muscle*, a jaw depressor with two bellies, which is attached between the mastoid process and inferior border of body of mandible (the digastric fossa); (2) *geniohyoid*, which elevates or moves the hyoid bone forwards or backwards depending on how the hyoid bone is fixed and is attached between the inferior genial tubercles and the hyoid body; (3) *mylohyoid*, an elevator or depressor the hyoid bone depending on the activity in surrounding muscles, *which is* attached between the hyoid and the mylohyoid line; and (4) *stylohyoid*, a retractor, elevator or stabiliser of the hyoid bone, which is attached between the styloid process and the hyoid bone.

7. *Jaw Opening and Closing Cycle Combining the Supra- and Inframandibular Muscles*

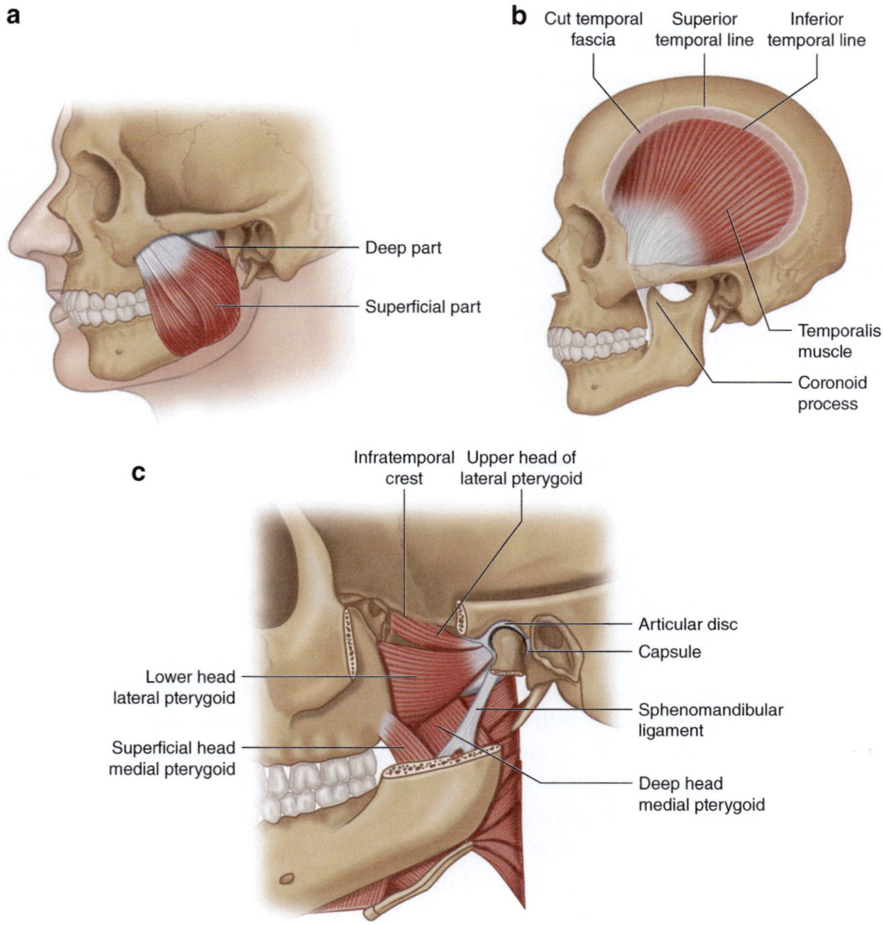

Fig. 2 Muscles of mastication

The process of jaw opening is a series of events occurring in the manner described below that combines the actions of the supra- and inframandibular muscles.

- Temporalis, masseter and medial pterygoid relax—the jaw essentially drops a short distance under gravity.
- A pure hinge movement occurs, opening the jaw very slightly.
- Lateral pterygoid pulls and protracts the jaw slightly—this allows the jaw to drop further under gravity as it is pulled clear of its anterior (articular tubercle) and posterior (parotid) limitations.
- Protraction and depression under gravity continues in a steeples cycle over the normal jaw opening range.
- The inframandibular muscles (digastric and suprahyoid muscles) are active at the extremes of movement.

The process of jaw elevation is essentially a reversal of jaw opening. Here, the lateral pterygoid relaxes first, and temporalis, masseter and medial pterygoid contract together to raise the mandible. The posterior and middle fibres pull upwards and may pull backwards to locate the condyle in the fossa.

8. *Neurovascular Supply*

The primary vascular supply to the TMJ is via the superficial temporal artery laterally and the maxillary artery medially. Additionally, penetrating vessels supplying the lateral pterygoid muscle supply the mandibular head. Venous drainage of the anterior aspect of the joint and is to the pterygoid venous plexus. The retrodiscal structures have an associated rich neurovascular (predominantly venous) plexus on the posterior aspect; the plexus is emptied and filled by pressure produced by the alternating anterior and posterior movements of the jaw, where the mandibular condyle shunts blood from one region to the other. The neurovascular nature of the retrodiscal structures is what causes substantial acute pain when a disc is displaced without reduction in the early phases, but it is also what most likely helps the disc remodel and form a pseudodisc in the subsequent 12–18 months. Lymph from the joint region drains into the deep upper cervical lymph nodes around the internal jugular vein.

With regard to the innervation of the region, it is worth noting that the articular tissues and the dense part of the disc are devoid of innervation. The sensory innervation of the tissues associated with the capsular ligament and looser part of the articular disc are supplied via the auriculotemporal nerve, a branch of the mandibular division of the trigeminal nerve (CN V3) and masseteric nerves as well as through postganglionic sympathetic nerves. The TMJ capsule, the lateral temporomandibular ligament and tissue behind the articular surfaces have within them both nociceptors and mechanoceptors. The latter aid in proprioceptive sensation for controlling mandibular movement and posture. Several of the nerves innervating the joint may be vasosensory and vasomotor and may further be involved in synovial fluid production.

The masticatory muscles are innervated by the motor division of the mandibular division of the trigeminal nerve which sits deep within the infratemporal fossa. The nerve travels into the region through the foramen ovale from its trifurcation within the middle cranial fossa and divides into two main divisions (anterior and posterior) within the infratemporal fossa. The anterior division of this branch of the tripart nerve is mainly motor and gives branches to all the muscles of mastication, with the exception of medial pterygoid muscle, which receives its innervation from a separate nerve off the main stem of the mandibular division of the trigeminal nerve, the medial pterygoid nerve (the SPAMM acronym is a useful guide—*Sensory mainly Posterior, Anterior mainly Motor bar Medial pterygoid*). The anterior division also provides a sensory branch, the buccal nerve (formally known as the long buccal nerve), which traverses the skin overlying buccinator and is important in dental anaesthesia. The posterior division of the mandibular division of the trigeminal nerve subdivides into the sensory lingual and inferior alveolar nerves. Both of these are of considerable importance clinically. They pass between the medial pterygoid muscle and ramus of the mandible in the pterygomandibular space. The lingual nerve passes forwards to the floor of the mouth and supply sensation to the anterior two-thirds of the tongue. A motor branch (nerve to mylohyoid) from the inferior alveolar supplies the mylohyoid and anterior digastric muscles. The inferior alveolar nerve itself enters the mandible via the mental foramen to innervate the mandibular teeth, the anatomy of which enables almost complete anaesthesia of the mandibular teeth with one procedure.

9. *Functions of the Joint*

The functional movements of the joint are elevation (anterior and middle fibres of temporalis, superficial and deep fibres of masseter and medial pterygoid), depression (lateral pterygoids aided by the digastric, geniohyoid and mylohyoid muscles), protraction (lateral and medial pterygoids) and retraction (posterior fibres of temporalis aided by the digastric and geniohyoid muscles). The functional movement of elevation and depression is the result of the combination of hinge and translation movements. Initially, a small hinge movement occurs, after which depression occurs further and thereafter forward translation movement. Translation is needed as movement is limited by the articular tubercle and parotid gland.

At rest, the mandibular head is separated from the mandibular fossa by a thick posterior band. As the head moves forwards, it becomes associated with the thinner parts of the disc. The head moves in an arc, its axis of rotation near the lingula. The articular disc only moves about half the distance of the condyle. Elevation reverses the process. Protraction and retraction are nearly pure translation movements.

It is only during "the power stroke of mastication" that jaw muscles exert large forces, even though they are capable of doing so even otherwise. The prime function of the mandible, however, is to exert the required force for breaking down food to aid digestion. It does this via the teeth. Lateral movements of the mandible create a shear component of force that potentiates "the power stroke of mastication". The TMJ can accommodate sliding and rotation in the parasagittal plane. The sliding movement is possible as the capsular ligament surrounding the upper joint compartment is loose, but the same ligament enclosing the lower joint compartment is tight. As a result, the mandibular condyle can only rotate over the depression inside the articular disc that is formed inside the annulus.

4 Understanding Pain

4.1 What Is Pain, and What Is It For?

Pain is a useful and adaptive phenomenon. It helps make us aware of when our bodies are being damaged or potentially damaged. It also limits function, thereby facilitating the healing process. However, an injury, disease, lesion or even prolonged stimulation of the sensory nervous system can lead to persistent pain, which serves no protective function and can negatively impact a person's physical, social and psychological wellbeing.

4.2 Nociception Versus Pain

Nociception is the mechanism of processing information about noxious stimuli at the level of the neuron. Consider nociception similar to a computer connecting to the Internet, with messages constantly being communicated within the body (Internet), which cannot be seen or felt, but which can be objectively measured (as the number of messages and size of messages). Pain, however, is what we actually feel (using the Internet example: what the user sees on the screen) and is defined as "an unpleasant sensory and emotional experience associated with, or resembling that associated with, actual or potential tissue damage" [3]. What this means is that pain is a complex output created by the central nervous system (CNS). The body listens to all the nociceptive input, to which it adds sensory information such as what it is seeing, for example: "That looks like a deep cut". It reflects on previous experience: "How did it feel the last time I cut myself?" Finally, it considers the individual's current state: "The body is tired therefore less able to cope with injury at present". From all this information, the body outputs what we feel as pain, making pain a subjective and personal experience.

These nociceptive mechanisms can be manipulated pharmacologically in order to reduce an individual's experience of pain. Pain can also be reduced through psychosocial management resulting in the pain "output" being lower despite nociceptive "input" being unchanged. The distinction between nociception and pain is essential, particularly when considering the social and psychological components of pain and its impact on a person.

4.3 The Process of Nociception

Nerve fibres which transmit information about fine, discriminative touch possess specialised receptors. However, neurones which carry noxious signals have free nerve endings called nociceptors which do not have any specialised structure. Nociceptors respond to different stimuli, for example, intense mechanical stimuli, hot or cold, or the presence of substances present in damaged tissues. Nociceptors may be polymodal, responding to several stimuli whilst others respond only to one. As Fig. 3a demonstrates, many substances are released within damaged tissues such as potassium and hydrogen ions, serotonin (5-HT), histamine, bradykinin, prostaglandins (e.g. PGE_2), interleukins (e.g. IL-1β) and leukotrienes, and these algogenic (pain-causing) substances can either stimulate nociceptors directly or sensitise them by lowering their threshold to responding to other stimuli.

When stimulated above their activation threshold, nociceptors generate action potentials which travel along the axon towards the central nervous system. Two

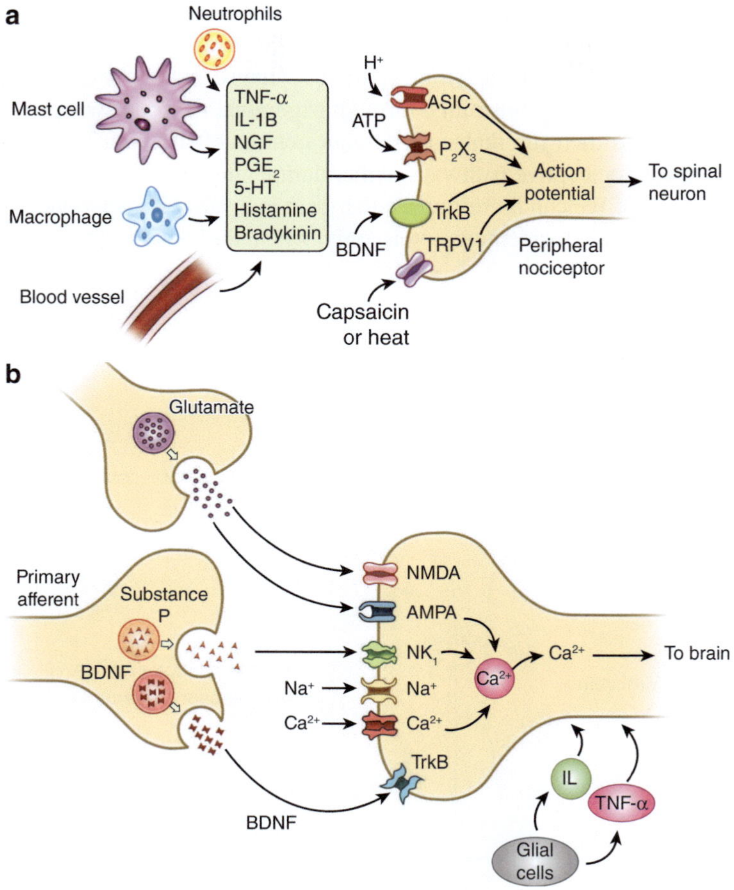

Fig. 3 Peripheral and central sensitisation. Notes: (**a**) Peripheral sensitisation and (**b**) central sensitisation. *Abbreviations:* AMPA α-Amino-3-hydroxy-5-methyl-4-isoxazolepropionic acid receptor, ATP adenosine triphosphate, ASIC acid-sensing ion channels, BDNF brain-derived neurotropic factor, CGRP calcitonin gene-related peptide, 5-HT 5-hydroxytryptamine (serotonin), IL interleukin, NMDA N-methyl-D-aspartate receptor, NGF nerve growth factor, PG prostaglandin, NK_1 neurokinin-1, TNF tumour necrosis factor, TrkB tyrosine receptor kinase B, TRPV transient receptor potential vanilloid receptor

types of fibres transmit noxious signals in the orofacial region: small diameter, unmyelinated c fibres which transmit their signals relatively slowly and the faster transmitting, lightly myelinated and comparatively larger diameter Aδ fibres. When we injure ourselves, an immediate sharp pain is first felt due to mechanical or thermal stimulation of Aδ fibres; this is followed by the slower, more sustained aching pain transmitted by c fibres in response to substances released in damaged tissues. These phenomena are termed first pain and second pain, respectively, and appear to be represented differently at the level of the cerebral cortex, suggesting that they may serve different biological functions [2].

Nociceptive signals are not simply transmitted unchanged along the trigemino-thalamic pathways (Fig. 4) from the periphery to the central nervous system (CNS), instead signals are modified each time neurones synapse on their path to the cerebral cortex. Orofacial pain is transmitted through trigeminal neurones which synapse in the brainstem and then the thalamus. Higher centres of the brain can modify the signals sent via nociceptive pathways, either dampening or potentiating their transmission (Fig. 3b). We can therefore see that pain is a variable experience, which is quite separate from nociception—it is only when these nociceptive signals are

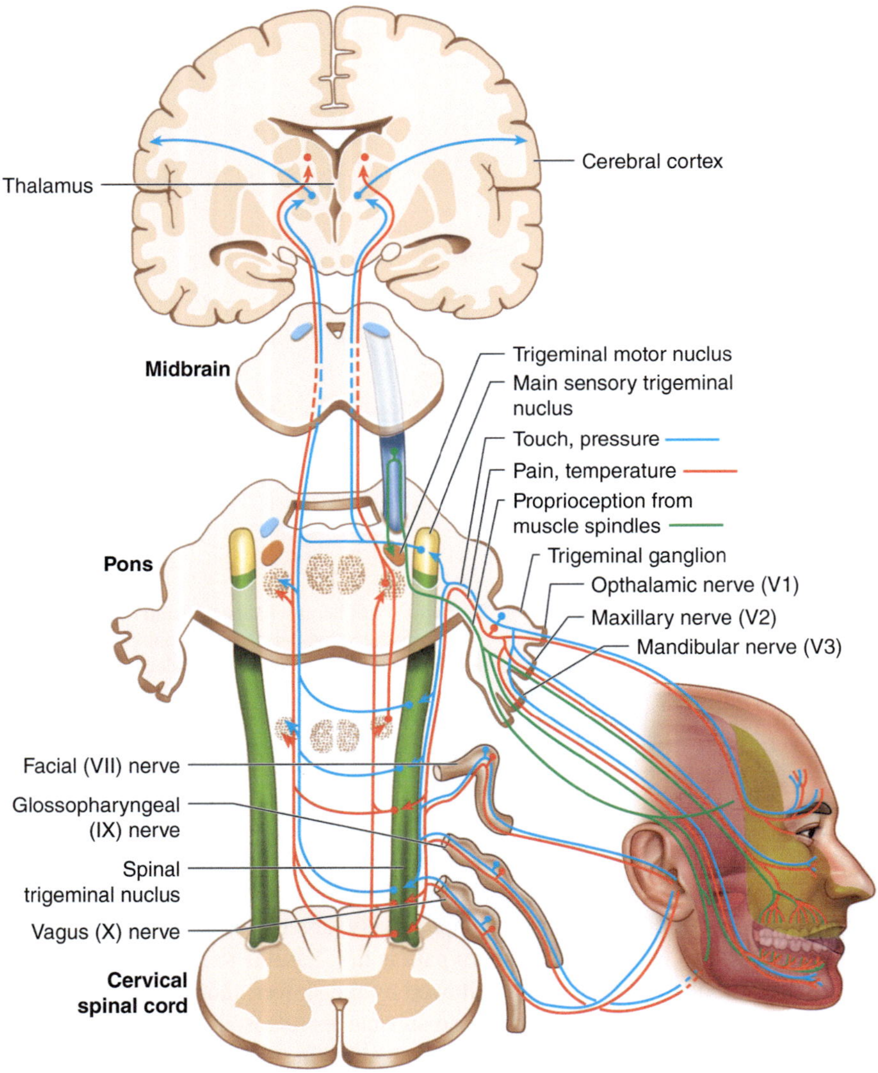

Fig. 4 Trigeminothalamic pathways

integrated in the cerebral cortex with all the other available information for that individual at that time that pain is experienced.

4.4 Nociceptive Pathways

The temporomandibular joint (TMJ), muscles of mastication and associated structures are innervated by both Aδ and c fibres. Afferent fibres (those travelling from the periphery to the central nervous system) project from the periphery to the pons in the brainstem via the trigeminal ganglion (although neurones do not synapse here) as shown in Fig. 4. After entering the pons in the brainstem, afferent fibres carrying pain and temperature signals synapse with second-order neurons in the spinal trigeminal nucleus. Some mechanical nociceptors are not activated under normal physiological movements but will send signals in extremes of mandibular movement. It is possible that the reduced threshold for activation seen in peripheral sensitisation, discussed below, results in these neurones depolarising during the "normal" range of movement, thus causing pain. Under normal conditions, Aδ fibres are the fibres which most commonly send nociceptive signals as they are more easily able to overcome their firing threshold. However, chemical stimulation leads to greater firing of c fibres which have higher mechanical thresholds for depolarisation.

Second-order neurons ascend from the spinal trigeminal nucleus and cross over to the contralateral side of the brainstem before ascending further to the thalamus, which is the major relay in the brain for all incoming sensory information. These fibres synapse with third-order neurons in the thalamus, before projecting to their final destination in sensory areas of the cerebral cortex. Interestingly, a new pathway has been identified in mice in which first-order nociceptive neurons synapse directly with brain areas related to emotion, anxiety and threat (the limbic system) [4]. This direct circuit may explain why orofacial pain is more emotionally loaded and impactful, with increased suffering and fear compared to pain experienced elsewhere in the body [5].

4.5 Mechanisms of Peripheral Sensitisation

Injured tissues and surrounding healthy tissues often become uncomfortable when subjected to stimuli, such as light touch, which would not usually cause pain: for example, the discomfort of wearing clothing over sunburnt skin. Substances present at the site of injury activate nociceptors directly, but they also sensitise or "wake up" other neurones which do not normally respond to stimuli in the absence of these substances. These silent nociceptors begin sending nociceptive signals in response to mechanical or thermal stimulation. Additionally, the threshold of nociceptors sensitised by these algogenic substances is lowered, and the area of tissue to which they respond (their receptive field) is increased. The net result is that more nociceptive input is sent to the CNS for the same physical stimulus, meaning that painful stimuli are perceived as more painful (hyperalgesia) and stimuli which would not usually produce pain begin to do so (allodynia), with all of this occurring over an area greater than the site of the injury itself; these processes contribute to peripheral sensitisation depicted in Fig. 3a. In the initial stages of injury, peripheral sensitisation serves as a protective mechanism which limits movement and function to allow healing to occur; however if prolonged, peripheral sensitisation can contribute to persistent pain after healing has occurred.

Aside from algogenic substances released from injured tissue, neurones themselves contribute to peripheral sensitisation. When action potentials are generated in nociceptive neurones, these propagate not only towards the CNS but also in the opposite direction towards the periphery and along other branches of the same nerve fibre. These potentials stimulate the release of substances from the neurone (neuropeptides) which activate and sensitise other nociceptors, thus contributing to peripheral sensitisation. Neurones themselves also become altered as a result of peripheral sensitisation; for example, the expression of a certain type of voltage-gated sodium channel involved in pain sensation ($Na_v1.7$) appears to increase in trigeminal nociceptive neurones in painful states, potentially contributing to sensitisation of neurones in the peripheral nervous system.

4.6 Mechanisms of Central Sensitisation

Sensitisation also occurs at the level of the trigeminal ganglion and centrally in the CNS at the trigeminal nucleus and beyond. Although central sensitisation contributes to neuronal healing, it is also strongly linked to the development of persistent pain states. The early response to peripheral inflammation in the trigeminal ganglion is the release of inflammatory cytokines, shown in Fig. 3b. This causes proliferation of satellite (e.g. glial) cells and can lead to further inflammatory cytokine release. At the same time, the stimulus leads to NMDA receptor upregulation in neurons in the trigeminal ganglion, along with the release of neuropeptides such as CGRP and substance P, which lower the activation threshold of neurons increasing the likelihood of an action potential. The result of these changes is not only neuronal hyperexcitability, but the “soup” of inflammatory mediators affects adjacent neurons in the ganglion and explains the increased receptive field, the phenomenon of referred pain and the presence of mechanical and thermal allodynia seen in orofacial pain.

Mechanisms of sensitisation in the trigeminal nucleus within the brainstem are similar to those seen in the trigeminal ganglion, except that synaptic transmission is also affected through lowering the activation threshold of second-order neurons. When these processes are taken into account, it is not difficult to appreciate how central sensitisation can contribute to the symptoms of persistent pain often seen in TMD.

5 What Happens in Persistent Pain

To fully understand how pain works, it is also important to understand why we experience pain. In 1979, Patrick Wall described pain as a motivational state with functions to promote protective behaviours and those associated with help-seeking and rest in order to promote escape and healing [6].

As discussed, it has been widely acknowledged within the scientific literature for over 20 years that all pain is created in the brain. Nociceptive signals from the body are often highly relevant to creating pain in the brain and may be the major trigger for pain, but this is still dependent on context and on interpretation within the brain. This fact can be illustrated by two historically documented cases and with many everyday experiences. In 1995, a letter in *The British Medical Journal* (*The BMJ*) described the case of a construction worker who had jumped from a height and landed on a nail which was sticking up through a plank [1]. The nail pierced the worker's boot and immediately caused excruciating pain which remained until he was admitted to hospital, at which point he was sedated. The boot was cut from the patient's foot. To everybody's surprise, there was no injury, the nail having passed through the gap between the worker's toes. The pain, in this case, had been generated by the brain in the context of extremely strong external cues of serious injury. The converse may also occur where actual injury is present; Wall [6] reported a personal experience of being injured by a blow to the head which caused no pain until he realised the extent of his bleeding. It is common for injuries sustained whilst playing sport, for example, to cause little pain initially even if later found out to be quite serious.

These examples can best be explained by the understanding that pain is *not* an accurate description of damage to the body. As discussed earlier, pain is an output of the brain, taking into account all available information, including nociceptive signals and a vast range of contextual factors. In the case of acute pain (pain of up to 3 months duration), very often, injury and the associated nociception are the primary drivers of pain. As injury heals, the link between pain and nociception becomes weaker. At this stage, many other factors become important to the pain experience (see chapter "Psychological Considerations").

It would be a mistake to assume that the absence of visible injury means that there should be no pain or that pain is "psychological". This outdated view is more consistent with an erroneous understanding that pain is a description of physical damage. It is important to remember that pain is always generated in the brain and its function is to act as an alert. Nociceptive messages can only convey the message that something *may* be wrong. Our automatic processing systems in the brain then use other contextual information to determine what is happening and the best course of action.

Persistent pain (pain lasting for >3 months duration) can be likened to a burglar or car alarm that has been set to too sensitive a setting. In this case, the alarm (pain) will be triggered frequently, but the problem is with the settings of the alarm system itself rather than the presence of an intruder (injury); additionally, the ringing alarm is certainly real, and not imagined or "psychological". As discussed in chapter "Psychological Considerations", a host of factors can be involved in sensitising and maintaining this response, and there is variation between individuals. Unfortunately, if the alarm is loud and frequently triggered, the impact is often to increase focus on the problem (pain) at the expense of valued life activities and goals.

5.1 Explaining Persistent Pain to an Individual with TMD

For individuals suffering with TMD, persistent pain is often a difficult feature of their condition. Being told that they have pain with no damage to their body can feel confusing. Equally, it is challenging for clinicians who are also used to thinking about pain primarily as an indication of damage or infection. Clinicians may frequently be asked to "find the problem" because the patient understandably wants someone to "fix" their pain.

Explaining persistent pain to patients in a way that they can understand can be difficult [7]. It can be helpful initially to discuss elements of the pain as relating to "a jaw problem" which links to management strategies such as oral exercises and perhaps a splint, accompanied also by "a pain problem". This can then enable further discussion about the need to include management strategies that aim to calm the overactive nervous system that is contributing to the heightened experience of pain.

Patients at this stage, especially if they have a history of multiple interactions with healthcare professionals where they may have been dismissed, will frequently be sensitive to interpreting such explanations as meaning that their pain is not being recognised or validated or that the practitioner believes that their pain is "in their head". It is important therefore to state very clearly that you recognise the intensity of their pain and its impact. Since explanations of persistent pain and how it works are unfamiliar to most people, it may take several visits or conversations before they fully understand the nature of this type of pain and the importance of tailoring management strategies to it.

Discussing the nature of the patient's pain is often helpful in facilitating their understanding that the issue is with the pain system and not (or not only) with the jaw or related structures. For example, for some patients with persistent TMD, their pain often varies in presentation and severity from day to day: on some days, the jaw aches when they wake; on other days, it hurts when they chew, and sometimes, it does both. The location of their pain may vary, with the pain sometimes feeling like earache and on other days affecting the teeth. Patients may be reassured by explaining that this changing pattern does not fit with pain caused by one particular site of injury, such as a problematic tooth or a broken finger, whereby symptoms may be more consistent, and the location of the pain is less likely to vary.

Allodynia (pain caused by stimuli which don't usually cause pain) is another feature of persistent pain which if present can be explained to the patient to support understanding. Allodynia is often described by individuals presenting with TMD; for example, "My jaw pain is worse when I lie down a night and my cheek touches the pillow". We know that lying on a pillow is not damaging and should not usually cause pain, but the sensitised nervous system fires off warning signal to that gentle pressure which the brain perceives as pain.

One way of explaining complex constructs such as sensitisation is to describe a scenario that most people will be familiar with in everyday life. An example is that of a "stubbed" toe: usually, this occurs to just one small area, but often the toe goes red and is also painful in areas where you didn't hit it. This is a normal process, known as (peripheral) sensitisation, where the volume switch is turned up on the pain system to help protect the area and aid healing. As the toe starts to heal, the redness disappears first, but some pain remains in areas that are no longer red and weren't hit. This too is normal and an aspect of the sensitisation process. On some occasions however, sensitisation can continue well beyond the time when tissues are healed. Different, brain-related (central) mechanisms also become involved and maintain the high sensitivity even though it is no longer adaptive. In other words, the "pain alarm" becomes stuck on a highly sensitive setting in order to protect an area of the body, even in the absence of the need for such a high level of protection, or after the problem that caused that need has resolved. We know that the capacity for this type of brain adaptability is present in everyone. We are also starting to understand how some factors serve to enhance it and make it more likely that the pain persists longer than "normal".

Sensitisation in persistent TMD can therefore be described to patients using a combination of the analogy of the car alarm as above, or a volume switch, which in their case is turned up to maximum for their pain system, and examples of normal experiences where sensitisation is commonly experienced. Following such discussions, it is always important to return to a summary of their relevance to the presenting problem. For most patients with persistent pain, the key messages are that their pain is real, believed and valid and that it is more than simply a structural problem. Management strategies, including self-management that aim to calm the nervous system, are therefore an important part of the picture.

References

1. Fisher JP, Hassan DT, Connor NO. Minerva. BMJ. 1995;310(6971):70.
2. Ploner M, Gross J, Timmermann L, Schnitzler A. Cortical representation of first and second pain sensation in humans. Proc Natl Acad Sci. 2002;99(19):12444–8.
3. Raja SN, Carr DB, Cohen M, Finnerup NB, Flor H, Gibson S, Keefe FJ, Mogil JS, Ringkamp M, Sluka KA, et al. The revised International Association for the Study of Pain definition of pain: concepts, challenges, and compromises. Pain. 2020;161(9):1976–82.
4. Rodriguez E, Sakurai K, Xu J, Chen Y, Toda K, Zhao S, Han BX, Ryu D, Yin H, Liedtke W, et al. A craniofacial-specific monosynaptic circuit enables heightened affective pain. Nat Neurosci. 2017;20(12):1734–43.
5. Schmidt K, Forkmann K, Sinke C, Gratz M, Bitz A, Bingel U. The differential effect of trigeminal vs. peripheral pain stimulation on visual processing and memory encoding is influenced by pain-related fear. Neuroimage. 2016;134:386–95.
6. Wall PD. On the relation of injury to pain. The John J. Bonica lecture. Pain. 1979;6(3):253–64.
7. Sekhon S. How to explain central sensitization to patients. 2020. [accessed 30/08/2022]. https://www.pathways.health/how-to-explain-central-sensitization-to-patients/.

Examination and Diagnosis of Temporomandibular Disorders

Stephen Davies and Emma Beecroft

1 Why Examine the Articulatory System?

To introduce this chapter, it is sensible to ask and answer the question, "Why would we wish to examine the articulatory system in TMD?" Whilst TMD do not wholly arise from the articulatory system, they can be responsible for dysfunction or pain within it. Hence, the ability to examine this orofacial system is important to any dental care professional who wishes to be able to diagnose and manage a TMD. It comprises of the temporomandibular joint and associated structures, the muscles of mastication and the occlusion.

This chapter describes a systematic approach to examination the articulatory system for all dental care professionals. This quick and easy examination protocol should be sufficient to diagnose the 12 most common TMD which fall under the broad groupings of:

1. Myogenous (muscular) disorders
2. Arthrogenous (intra-articular disorders)
    (a) Disc displacements
    (b) Degenerative joint disease

S. Davies (✉)
Division of Dentistry, University of Manchester, Manchester, UK
e-mail: stephen.j.davies@manchester.ac.uk

E. Beecroft
School of Dental Sciences, Newcastle University, Newcastle upon Tyne, UK
e-mail: Emma.beecroft@newcastle.ac.uk

S. Davies et al. (eds.), *Temporomandibular Disorders in Primary Dental Care*, BDJ Clinician's Guides, https://doi.org/10.1007/978-3-032-01301-9_3

   (c) Arthralgia
   (d) Subluxation

3. Headache attributed to TMD

The ability to examine the articulatory system is an essential skill for dental care professionals who wish to be able to diagnose and manage TMD.

It is suggested that an examination of the articulatory system is completed:

- For every new patient in order *to screen for a TMD*
- When a patient complains of non-odontogenic pain in order *to avoid diagnostic bias*
- Prior to major restorative, orthodontic or surgical treatment *in order to avoid exacerbating a pre-existing TMD*

The reasons why a protocol for examining the articulatory system might be useful are clear.

Firstly, individuals living with TMD deserve as contemporaneous and as comprehensive care as patients with other dental or facial problems that present to healthcare professionals. Diagnosis and management of these conditions are, at least initially, the responsibility of our profession and ideally will start in primary care.

Secondly and within the discipline of restorative dentistry, it can impact on the success of a restorative course of treatment if the patient has a pre-existing TMD or develops one during treatment. Furthermore, because the examination of the articulatory system can include an occlusal analysis, it will be very useful whether the treatment is being provided to either the confirmative or re-organised approaches.

Finally, the ability to exclude a diagnosis of TMD is important. Too often, patients are referred into a TMD clinic because a dental care professional cannot find the cause of a patient's facial pain so, the assumption is made: "It must be a TMD problem". Once it has been established through an articulatory system examination that TMD is an unlikely diagnosis, further investigations will become indicated to progress the diagnostic process. If a dental care professional is unable to diagnose TMD, it follows that they will also be unable to exclude TMD as a cause of the same patient's complaint.

Importantly, several conditions present with symptoms which mimic TMD, a small number of which (<1%) represent neoplastic pathologies [1, 2]. Table 1 displays "Red Flag" clinical findings in history or examination and their possible origin that clinicians should be aware of. The detection of any such finding should be investigated in detail, and urgent referral to appropriate general medical or secondary care services should be processed.

Table 1 TMD Red flags adapted from [3]

Sign	Possible cause or origin
History of previous malignancy with facial pain or headache	Potential for new primary, recurrence or metastases
Swelling, mass or lymphadenopathy	Neoplastic, infective or autoimmune
Sudden and unplanned weight loss	Neoplastic, systemic illness
Pyrexia	Infective
Neurological signs/symptoms Acute onset sensory change (smell, hearing, vision) Motor or sensory function changes	Neoplastic, infective or autoimmune cause
Persistent nasal bleeding or (purulent) discharge	Neoplastic (nasopharyngeal) or infective
Acute onset, substantial or deteriorating trismus	Neoplastic, infective or traumatic cause
Persistent hoarse voice (≥3 weeks) or dysphagia	Neoplastic, infective
Persistent mouth ulcer(s) (≥3 weeks)	Neoplastic
Occlusal changes	Neoplastic, traumatic, growth disturbance
Cramp like pain and weakness of the jaw (claudication), visual disturbances, temporal arteries palpably engorged and inflamed, headache, trismus	Giant cell arteritis
New onset jaw pain in those taking bisphosphonates or related medication	Risk of medication related osteonecrosis of the jaws

2 Suggested Protocols

Before moving on to objective assessment, namely, the examination of the patient, it is worth considering how to record the patient's subjective narrative or history. It is important to note that whilst most texts talk about "taking a history" from the patient, it is more collegiate and conducive to remember to work in partnership with patients to discuss this process in terms of "receiving the history".

3 A Guide to Receiving a History from a TMD Patient

Histories in TMD can be difficult, especially if the person recounting the history has had pain for a long time with multiple visits or treatments. A sensible approach is to:

- Try to write the history in an orderly way. Often patients will tell their story in a disorderly narrative. The use of the *SOCRATES* (*S*ite, *O*nset, *C*haracter, *R*adiation, *A*ssociated symptoms, *T*ime, *E*xacerbating/relieving factors, *S*everity) pain assessment tool can help structure pain history taking.
- Identify if there is more than one complaint, e.g. facial pain and headache, and make your notes under "Pain 1: Facial pain" and "Pain 2: Headache". This will help you ascertain if there are two comorbid conditions or one condition causing two presentations of pain.

- Be empathetic but maintain control of the history being given. For example: ask the patient to focus on one complaint at a time; gently interject to clarify or use the patient's own terms to explain/summarise understanding thus far; complete the history, and if you've run out of time, consider bringing the patient back for an examination as soon as possible by explaining you have now got a good idea of the problem and its history and that this is very important but need sufficient time to conduct a thorough examination (Box 1).

Box 1: An example of a patient history-taking proforma

Guidelines on Taking a History for a TMD Patient
Patient's Aspiration
What has brought you here?
What are you hoping we can do for you?

Presenting Complaint

1. <u>PAIN</u>

Site
Do they point to the area of the TMJ? Do they point to the muscles of mastication?
May be a face and head diagram?

Onset/Event
Is it a long standing problem? Did it start in time of stress? Did something specific happen to precipitate it?

Character
Sharp shooting pain? Ache? Throbbing

Radiation
Does the pain stay localised or does it spread.

Associations
Is the pain associated with a click? Or a grating sound in the joint? Is it associated with limited opening?

Timing
When waking in the morning? Following heavy chewing?

Exacerbating/relieving factors
Anything that makes it worse, e.g. heavy chewing, yawning, habits, stress, cold?
Anything that makes it better, e.g. holidays, previous treatments given?

Severity
On a scale of 1–10, how bad is the pain? Is it like that all the time, or does it get better/worse?

(continued)

Box 1 (continued)

Does This Pain Affect Your State of Mind or Mood?
If YES: Give PHQ4 to Patient to complete.

2. **NOISES?**

Type of Noise Clicking Grating [Crunching Grinding]
Consistent or Intermittent? If intermittent, can you open normally when No Noise?
Onset/Event
History
Any Association Between Noise and Pain?

3. **LIMITED OPENING?**

If patient describes a LOCK, is it Open or Closed Lock?
Consistent or Intermittent?
If intermittent, is there a Click when you can open?
If Intermittent, How Long Does the Closed Lock Last: Seconds, Hours, Days?
Onset/Event
Did It Used to Click?
History
Any Association Between Noise and Pain?

4. **Do you sleep well ?**
5. **Is there anything that I should have asked you?**
6. **Medical History:**

Needs to be reviewed for relevant details, such as:
- History of arthritic conditions
- History of mental health diagnosis psychiatric problems including depression and anxiety
- History of neuropathic pain
- System pain conditions, e.g. fibromyalgia

4 An Examination Protocol

Figures 1 and 2 represent a comprehensive examination proforma for use in clinical practice, which includes all required examination elements as recommended by DC/TMD. The addition of the Trismus checklist, to support screening for the possibility of sinister mimicking pathology will be discussed further in the chapter [4]. Readers should be aware that adoption of the *brief* Diagnostic Criteria for TMD [*b*DC/TMD] [5] may result in a shortened version of this examination protocol in the future.

Reference	
Surname:	
Forename:	
Date of Birth:	

The 3-minute Articulatory System Exam

Date of exam	

Location:

STAFF NAME **GDC** **Signature**

Temporomandibular Joint		Right	Left
Tender to palpation?	*Lateral pole*		
	Causes Familiar PAIN		
Noises?	*Clicks*	Right Left Bilateral Soft Loud Consistent Intermittent [intermittent with .... Opening Closing Both Cycle: Early Mid Late Painful Painless Single Multiple	
	If patient has consistent clicks, do these clicks disappear when the patient opens from a protrusive mandibular position?		
	Crepitus	Right Left Bilateral Painful Painless	
Range of motion? (mm)	*Lateral*	R ← → L	
MAXIMUM MOUTH OPENING: _____mm	*Vertical*	Str Comfortable Maximal With Passive Stretch	

If this is less than 30mm, complete TRISMUS CHECKLIST below:

	Yes*	No
Opening less than 20 mm		
Progressively worsening trismus		
Absence of history of TMD related symptoms (incl. Clicking)		
Pain of Non-myofascial origin (neuralgia, etc)		
Swollen Lymph Glands		
Suspicious intra oral soft tissue lesion		
Older than 45 yrs		

* *If any of the answers are 'yes', see Trismus Checklist Flow Diagram and refer to OMFS*

Fig. 1 Comprehensive articulatory system examination proforma page 1. Includes TMJ noises, pain and range of motion

Muscle Tenderness *MARK ☐ IF Causes Familiar PAIN*

	Technique	Right	Left
Temporalis	Palpation		
Masseter	Palpation		
Lateral pterygoid	Resisted movement test		

Occlusion Record

Skeletal			
Angles			
Static occlusion	Does C.O occur in C.R?		
	If not – premature contact in C.R? *Roughly:* *or* *Exactly:* *Direction of slide from C.R to C.O:* Optional Vh ☐ vH ☐ *Freedom in centric occlusion?*		
Dynamic occlusion		Right	Left
	Non-working side interferences?		
	Working side interferences?		
	Crossover position: *Non-working side*		
	Working side		
	Canine guidance?		
	Group function?		

Excessive wear ☐ *Evidence of tooth/restoration fracture* ☐

Cheek ridging ☐ *tongue scalloping* ☐

Compression Test **Elicits Pre-Auricular Pain?**

Tongue Spatulae

	Pain on RHS?	Pain on LHS?
on RHS	☐ *myogenic*	☐ *arthrogenic*
on LHS	☐ *myogenic*	☐ *arthrogenic*

Fig. 2 Comprehensive articulatory system examination proforma page 2. Includes Muscular and occlusal examination proforma

The presented protocol fits onto two pages of A4 and takes an experienced clinician less than 5 minutes to complete. We will now talk clinicians through a comprehensive TMD clinical examination following the order of the presented proforma.

5 Examination of the Temporomandibular Joints

Without the option of specialised imaging techniques in most care settings [6], the clinical examination of the joints can be distilled down to four questions:

1. It the joint painful upon palpation?
2. Does it make noises?
3. Does it have a normal range of movement?
4. Is the joint painful upon load (compression test)?

It is worth noting that the use of plain radiographs has little diagnostic value for TMD and there are considerable dangers of confirmation bias or false positives. A radiograph has no value in determining condylar position [7].

5.1 It the Joint Painful upon Palpation?

It is easy to apply pressure to the lateral pole of the TMJ, because it lies very close to the skin. If it does prove to be tender to palpation, it needs to be recorded whether that pressure elicits the pain about which the patient is consulting us—so-called pain that is familiar to their complaint or “familiar pain”.

5.2 Does the TMJ Make Noises?

A click, which is single explosive noise, and crepitus, which is a continuous grating noise, are the two noises that the joint can make. Noises can be palpated and listened for during examination. As they can be sporadic and difficult to detect, positive finding of a joint noise can be documented if the patient reports its presence in the last 30 days [8]. Simply detecting a noise gives you limited information, whereas eliciting detailed information as to the type of noise, frequency of presentation, location and impact can help towards making a provisional diagnosis.

5.2.1 Crepitus

If crepitus is detected, the examination should identify which joint is affected and whether it occurs with or without pain. Crepitus is indicative of a TMD subdiagnosis of degenerative joint disease.

5.2.2 Intermittent Click

If clicks are intermittent with periods of a “hard endpoint”, then this is *suggestive that there is a disc displacement* which sometimes reduces (goes back to correct position) and sometimes does not (disc stays displaced). A displaced disc can cause limited jaw opening as the disc gets in the way of normal condylar rotation and slide movement. In such situations, the limited opening is described as a "hard endpoint trismus". The patient often feels a sensation of blockage to movement or the jaw being stuck in the pre-auricular region. In such situations, mouth opening cannot be increased by a clinician trying to actively stretch the mandible open. If there is <5 mm of passive stretch when the clinician tries to stretch the mouth opening and it feels like a "hard" object is resisting opening (there is no "give"), it suggests disc displacement without reduction and limited opening.

A useful way of helping the patient understand this question is to use an analogy: "Does it feel like you are trying to open door against a door stop [*hard endpoint*] or against someone holding the door shut [*soft endpoint*]?

If clicks are intermittent with periods of normal silent opening, then it is suggestive that there is not a permanently displaced disc, equating to disc displacement with reduction with intermittent locking.

It is important to understand that you can have a disc displacement without reduction which has no joint sounds.

5.2.3 Consistent Reproducible Click

A constant reproducible click is suggestive of a disc displacement with reduction [DDwR]. In the majority of cases, this condition may need no active treatment as it is very common in the asymptomatic population; less than one in three people note any progression to the disc staying out of position ("without reduction"). Management of TMD should not be initiated with the primary aim of changing joint noise. Joint noise without pain is effectively a normal anatomical variant which requires no treatment above reassurance and education.

If it is painful when the click occurs, it may be useful to note whether the click disappears if the patient opens from a more protrusive jaw relationship. In asking the patient to follow this manoeuvre, it is essential that they first open wide and then close to this protrusive mandibular position (close with their chin pushing forwards). This is prudent as simply pushing the mandible forward without first opening may not *recapture the disc*. It may push the disc further forward, making *recapture* less likely.

If the click disappears when the patient opens from a more protrusive mandibular position [for a Class I relationship, this would be from an edge-to-edge incisor relationship], then:

- Either at the moment when the click occurs there is a sudden sharp pain or if there are episodes of either disc displacement with reduction [DDwR] with intermittent locking or disc displacement without reduction [DDwoR] that are becoming more frequent and/or longer.
- And if the patient is willing to tolerate the significant imposition of wearing one, then an anterior repositioning splint [ARPS] may rarely be indicated. These appliances are best provided by clinicians with significant experience, and individuals using such appliances should be regularly reviewed to avoid irreversible occlusal changes. These are very difficult splints for a patient to tolerate [24 hours/day for 3 months]. In most cases of DDwoR or DDwR with intermittent locking, this treatment is worse than the condition.

5.3 Does the Joint Have a Normal Range of Movement?

Normal mouth opening determines how far the head of the condyle translates downwards, forwards and medially in the glenoid fossa; how to document such movement is shown in Fig. 3. It is important to note that "normal" mouth opening is heavily subjective and therefore dependent both on how you measure it as a clinician and the patient themselves. "Normal" can range from 35 to 55 mm of unassisted mouth opening, and lateral excursions can range between 7 and 12 mm. Judgements of decreased movement are therefore hard to achieve in an objective fashion, but <35 mm unassisted mouth opening would be considered restricted in most individuals as would <7 mm of lateral excursion.

It is important to remember that the joint does not move in a range you might consider "normal" for the patient and that the limitation to its movement may either be due to soft tissue, muscular guarding through pain or an intra-articular obstacle [e.g. a displaced non-reducing disc as discussed above]. For cases of muscular

a

Temporomandibular Joint		Right	Left
Tender to palpation?	*Lateral pole*		
	Causes Familiar PAIN		

b

Noises?	*Clicks*	Right Left Bilateral Soft Loud Consistent Intermittent [intermittent with .... Opening Closing Both Cycle: Early Mid Late Painful Painless Single Multiple
	If patient has consistent clicks, do these clicks disappear when the patient opens from a protrusive mandibular position?	
	Crepitus	Right Left Bilateral Painful Painless

c

Range of motion? (mm)	*Lateral*	R ⟵——⟶ L
MAXIMUM MOUTH OPENING: ______mm	*Vertical*	Str Comfortable Maximal With Passive Stretch
If this is less than 30mm, complete TRISMUS CHECKLIST		

Fig. 3 Examination of the temporomandibular joints

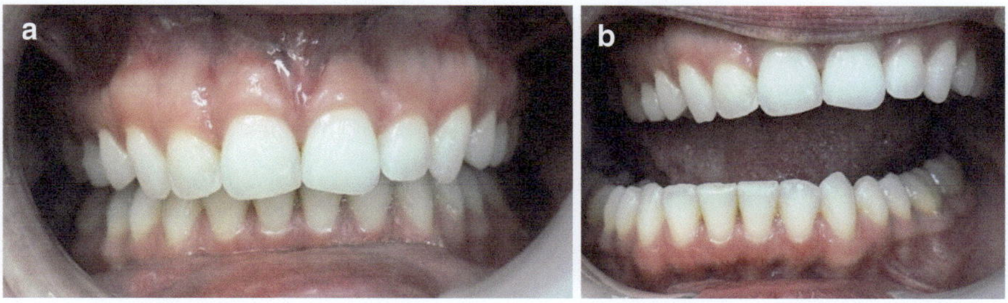

Fig. 4 Patient images displaying positive findings with regards to temporomandibular joint and occlusal examination. (**a**) Centric Occlusion, (**b**) Maximum Opening

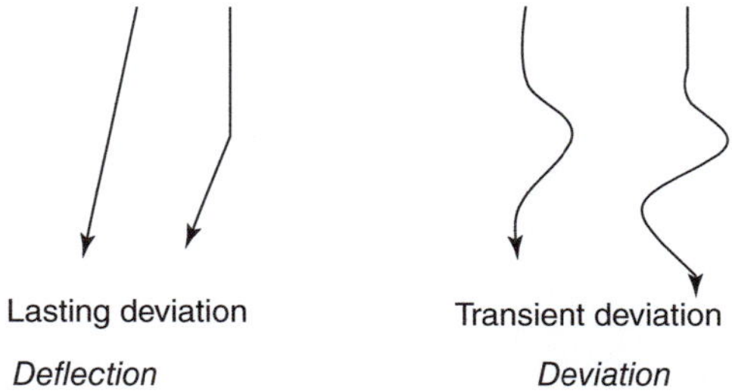

Fig. 5 In a Lasting Deviation the mandible goes off to one side, and stays on that side. In a Transient Deviation, the mandible goes of to one side but returns to the midline. The former is suggestive that one condyle is not translating as far as the other; in the later, they are translating an equal distance, but not at the same rate

guarding, passive stretch of mandibular opening by a clinician would be expected to increase mouth opening to at least partially overcome restriction and so that no "hard end point" resistance would be felt. As outlined above, a restricted opening with a consistent *hard end point* to the trismus is suggestive of an arthrogenous cause, most likely DDwoR, with limited opening.

A lasting deviation to one side is suggestive of a unilateral DDwoR (Fig. 5), whereas if the deviation is transient, i.e. returning to the midline, it probably means that both condyles are travelling to the same end points within the glenoid fossae but at different rates (Fig. 4).

If there is a consistent trismus of less than 30 mm, it should have triggered the "Trismus Checklist" [4] (Table 2). This is to flag up the possibility of an occult pathology being the cause of the limited opening; if any of the answers in this

Table 2 The Trismus Checklist: For completion in patient with reduced mouth opening (less than or equal to 30 mm passive opening)

	Yes	No
Inter-incisal opening <20 mm		
Progressively worsening trismus		
Absence of history of TMD-related symptoms (*incl.* clicking)		
Pain of non-myofascial origin (neuralgia, etc.)		
Swollen lymph glands		
Suspicious intra-oral soft tissue lesion		
Older than 45 years		
Difficulty swallowing		
Recent weight loss		
Neurological signs/symptoms Acute onset loss of smell or hearing Acute onset visual problems Neurosensory change Motor function changes		
If any of the answers are yes: Primary care setting: urgent oral and maxillofacial surgery referral Secondary care setting: urgent senior consultant assessment and urgent TMJ imaging as per senior consultant advice		

checklist are answered "Yes", [with the exception of a single "yes" to the question 'Older than 45 years'] then a dental care professional would be well advised to consider urgent referral to any oral and maxillofacial surgeon to investigate the possibility of a malignancy being the cause of the limited mouth opening [4, 9].

5.4 Is the Joint Painful on Load?

Pain in the pre-auricular region cannot not always be assumed to be coming from the TMJ; the lateral pterygoid is not only in the same region but is better innervated. A simple and quick test, the compression test, shown in Fig. 6, was developed by Mahan and Alling [10] to help differentiate between pre-auricular pain that has an arthrogenous and a myogenous origin.

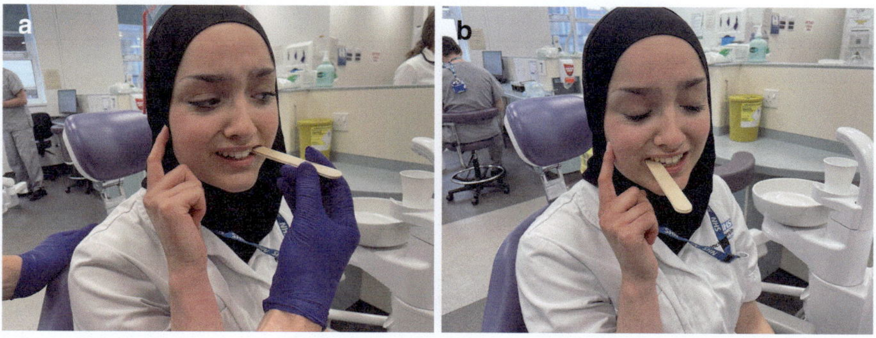

c

Compression Test
Tongue Spatulae

Elicits Pre-Auricular Pain?

	Pain on RHS?	**Pain on LHS?**
on RHS	☐ *myogenic*	☐ *arthrogenic*
on LHS	☐ *arthrogenic*	☐ *myogenic*

Fig. 6 **Compression test** Two-panel image showing a dental examination. In panel (**a**), a person is seated in a dental chair, with the clinician's gloved hand holding a wooden tongue spatula between the subject's clenched teeth on the LHS. The pained expression on their face indicates that discomfort is being experienced and their finger is pointing to the area over the TMJ on the RHS [contra-lateral] being the site of that discomfort, suggesting an arthrogenous pain in right TMJ. In panel (**b**), the same person is also experiencing discomfort, whist clenching on the tongue spatula. But now they are pointing to the muscles in their cheek region on the same side as they are clenching on the tongue spatula, suggesting a myogenous pain in the right masseter. Panel (**c**) shows exert of examination proforma page 2 (Fig. 2) focusing on documentation of compression test findings

5.5 Examination of the Muscles of Mastication

The first question when addressing this subject is whether examining muscles is a reliable test. In 2009 Kvåle et al., when examining the reliability of this test in general musculoskeletal pain, stated, "Palpation can be used in a reliable and valid way when screening patients with long-lasting pain", although some training was needed [11]. Many years previous to that study, Stockstill et al. stated, again with the caveat that of some operator expertise, "Muscle palpation is an important procedure in screening for TMD and assessing results of treatment outcome studies" [12].

There are four main masticatory muscles that are often discussed in examination protocols of the articulatory system (masseter, temporalis, medial and lateral pterygoid). The only muscles which are deemed to have an appropriate degree of sensitivity and specificity to support TMD examination are the masseter and temporalis, and examination should focus on assessing familiar pain, representative of the patient's complaint, in these two muscles.

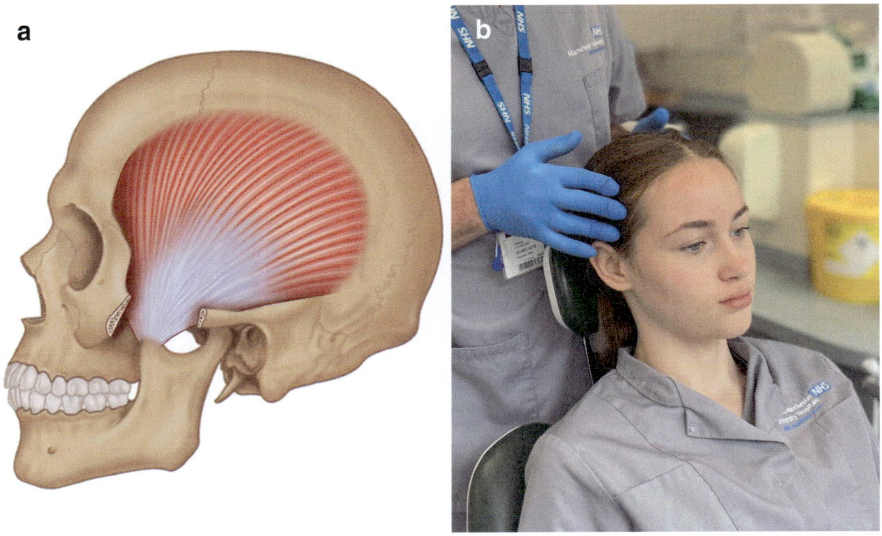

Fig. 7 **Temporalis** (**a**, **b**) Palpation of the temporalis muscles (**a**) anatomical drawing of the muscle; (**b**) clinical photos demonstrating palpation technique for temporalis

5.5.1 Temporalis Muscle

This fan-shaped muscle with fibres that run almost at right angle to each other is a very easy muscle to palpate because it is thin and overlays the flat hard surface of the cranium (Fig. 7a, b).

5.5.2 Masseter Muscle

Palpation of this muscle is also very easily done because it is possible for the operator to place a digit either side of it (Bimanual palpation) (Fig. 8a, b).

Palpation of each muscle should occur from superior to inferior and then posterior to anterior aspects to ensure the origin, body and insertion are all examined. In each of these muscle examinations, it must be recorded if there is pain and if this is a familiar pain to the patient's complaint and whether pain, if triggered, stays at the point of palpation (local myalgia), extends within the anatomical boundaries of the muscle (myofascial pain) or refers beyond the muscle being examined (myofascial pain with referral).

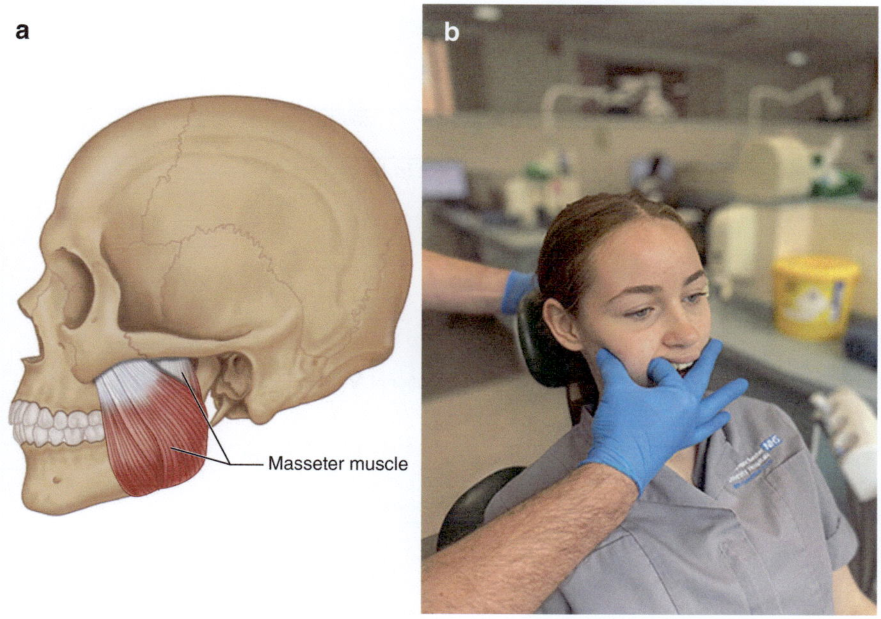

Fig. 8 Palpation of the masseter muscle: (**a**) anatomical drawing of muscle; (**b**) clinical photographs demonstrating bimanual palpation technique for the masseter muscle

5.6 Examination of the Occlusion

Occlusal records gathered using the suggested examination protocol will cover skeletal classification and static and dynamic occlusion, all of which may be affected and also influence treatment strategies for both TMD and any dental treatment which affected the occlusion (restorative dentistry or orthodontics) (Fig. 9).

Occlusion Record

Skeletal			
Angles			
Static occlusion	Does C.O occur in C.R?		
	If not – premature contact in C.R? *Roughly:* *or* *Exactly:* *Direction of slide from C.R to C.O:* Optional Vh ☐ vH ☐ *Freedom in centric occlusion?*		
Dynamic occlusion		**Right**	**Left**
	Non-working side interferences?		
	Working side interferences?		
	Crossover position: *Non-working side*		
	Working side		
	Canine guidance?		
	Group function?		

Excessive wear ☐ *Evidence of tooth/restoration fracture* ☐

Cheek ridging ☐ *tongue scalloping* ☐

Fig. 9 Occlusion Record

5.7 Other Examinations

Within the examination of the occlusion (Fig. 9), it is useful to record whether there is a history of excessive wear or fractured teeth, as an indication of trauma from occlusion which may or may not still be occurring. Soft tissue changes seen in the tongue and cheek mucosa may be an indication of a *current* bruxing habit [13]. It should be noted that bruxism is a spectrum from normal to pathological and cannot be definitively diagnosed without advanced instrumentation, e.g. polysomnography.

6 Diagnosis

Completion of a detailed clinical examination utilising the suggested protocol should result in clinical findings which can be used to inform a diagnosis. For the clinician, confirming the diagnosis is the point of clarity between exploration of symptoms, consolidation of clinical findings and the initiation of a management strategy. Clinically, diagnostic accuracy allows the appropriate management to be implemented and improves the patient's prognosis. For an individual living with TMD, diagnosis is often a more emotive concept. Being provided with a "name" for the condition which is causing their pain validates an individual's suffering, justifying their experience to themselves, their family, friends and work colleagues. It is the crucial first step towards acceptance and understanding and should ideally be provided at the point of first contact wherever possible. Delay in provision of diagnosis or lack of diagnostic certainty has been shown to influence both the intensity of TMD symptoms and their impact [14].

In 2014, Schiffman et al. [15] simplified diagnostic classification for TMD, confirming diagnostic terminology translatable for both research and clinical practice through the Diagnostic Criteria for Temporomandibular Disorders (DC/TMD). Under DC/TMD, TMD can be broadly classified as:

- *Myogenous* affecting muscles of mastication
- *Arthrogenous* involving the temporomandibular joint complex
- *Combination of the above*

The most common diagnosis on examination is the combination diagnosis of myalgia and arthralgia [8]. Table 3 displays the 12 most common TMD subtypes as

Table 3 Twelve most common TMD diagnostic subtypes shown in **bold**, linking clinical history and examination results to diagnosis. Luxation (*italicized*) is not one of the 12 most common subtypes but is included for completeness

Clinical history	Clinical examination findings	Specific findings related to pain or complaint	Diagnosis	Group
Pain in the jaw, temple, ear, or in front of the ear AND Pain modified with jaw movement, function or parafunction	Confirmation of pain in temporalis or masseter AND "Familiar" pain in masseter or temporalis produced during examination	Pain of muscular origin	**Myalgia**	Myogenous
		Pain localised to site of palpation	**Local myalgia**	
		Pain spreads beyond site of palpation but within the boundary of muscle	**Myofascial pain**	
		Pain reported at a site beyond the boundary of the muscle being palpated	**Myofascial pain with referral**	
Headache of any type in the temple AND Headache modified with jaw movement, function or parafunction	"Familiar" headache pain in the temple area produced during examination AND Confirmation of headache location in the area of temporalis muscles		**Headache attributed to TMD**	Headache

(continued)

Table 3 (continued)

Clinical history	Clinical examination findings	Specific findings related to pain or complaint	Diagnosis	Group
Any TMJ noise present with jaw movement or function in the last 30 days OR Patient reports any TMJ noise during exam (+/- TMJ pain)	Clicking, popping, or snapping detected during at least one of three repetitions of palpating the TMJ on opening/closing, lateral excursion, or protrusion	Joint noise but no locking	**Disc displacement with reduction**	Arthrogenous
Any TMJ noise present with jaw movement or function in the last 30 days OR Patient reports any TMJ noise during exam (+/- TMJ pain) AND Jaw locks with limited mouth opening, even for a moment, in the last 30 days		Jaw locks with limited mouth opening even for a moment then unlocks in the last 30 days	**Disc displacement with reduction with intermittent locking**	
Jaw locking so that mouth would not open all of the way AND Limitation in jaw opening severe enough to interfere with ability to eat	Maximum assisted opening with passive stretching less than 40 mm. The presence of TMJ noise on examination does not exclude this diagnosis		**Disc displacement without reduction with limited opening (i.e., "closed lock")**	
	Maximum assisted opening with passive stretching more than or equal to 40 mm. The presence of TMJ noise on examination does not exclude this diagnosis		**Disc displacement without reduction without limited opening**	
Any TMJ noise present with jaw movement or function in the last 30 days OR Patient reports any TMJ noise during exam (+/- TMJ pain)	Crepitus detected during examination		**Degenerative joint disease**	
Jaw locking or catching in a wide-open mouth position in the last 30 days, even for a moment, so it could not close from the wide-open position (+/- TMJ pain)	Positive finding of "open lock", which requires manipulation (self or clinician) to reduce	Self-manoeuvre required by patient to reduce dislocation	**Subluxation (i.e. "open lock")**	
		Clinician manoeuvre required to reduce dislocation	*Luxation (i.e. "open lock")*	
Pain in the jaw, temple, ear, or in front of the ear AND Pain modified with jaw movement, function or parafunction	Confirmation of pain in the area of the TMJ AND "Familiar" pain in the TMJ produced during examination		**Arthralgia**	

Adapted from Beecroft [16] based on information from Schiffman et al. [17]. *TMD* temporomandibular disorders, *TMJ* temporomandibular joint outlined by the DC/TMD and links these to their clinical presentation and examination findings. An understanding that TMD can be classified by sub-diagnosis is important, but not essential for successful initial management. In primary care situations, correctly identifying that an individual has myogenous, arthrogenous or a combination TMD (with myogenous and arthrogenous elements) is appropriate to inform appropriate management strategies and should be the focus.

The myogenous diagnoses include myalgia, local myalgia, myofascial pain and myofascial pain with referral. Myalgia (pain of muscular origin) is an overarching diagnosis, and the type of myalgia (local, myofascial pain and myofascial pain with referral) is separated through provocation testing on clinical examination of the muscles, resulting in specific finding related to pain complaint as highlighted in column 3 of Table 3.

The arthrogenous diagnoses include the four disc-displacement disorders, degenerative joint disease, subluxation and arthralgia. For disc displacements, pain elicited with function is often a result of the disc sitting anteriorly causing the retro discal tissue to stretch and move to a new position lying between the condylar head and articular eminence. As the retrodiscal tissue is well vascularised and contains nerve fibres, pressure, compression and movement on this tissue result in pain. Over time, this retro discal tissue will adapt, and a psuedo-disc will form, reducing pain and improving function, but the period of adaptation can be acutely painful.

Headache attributed to TMD is the final important sub-diagnosis to be aware of, and the prevalence of this secondary headache condition in orofacial pain clinics ranges from 5.4% to 29.3% [18, 19]. Headache attributed to TMD is more frequently associated with myogenous TMD than arthrogenous TMD and is significantly more prevalent with individuals with a concomitant primary headache diagnosis (e.g. migraine, tension-type headache) [20]. In a recent cross-sectional study consisting of participants with persistent myogenous TMD and a diagnosed primary headache condition, "61.6% of participants met the DC/TMD criteria for headache attributed to TMD" [21].

7 Less Common TMD Diagnoses

Table 4 provides taxonomic classification and brief description of some of the less common TMD, many of which are extremely rare and may not even be encountered by individuals in specialist orofacial pain practice.

Table 4 Taxonomic classification for temporomandibular disorders, not including the 12 most common TMD subtypes, i.e. rare TMD subtypes

Condition	Description
Hypomobility disorders	
Adhesions/Adherence	Fibrous adhesions present mainly in superior compartment of TMJ and result in decreased movement of disc condyle complex
Ankylosis (a) Fibrous	Widespread fibrotic changes in capsular ligaments with severely restrict joint movement
(b) Osseous	Bony proliferation which results in fusion of condyle to fossa, fusing bones of TMJ
Joint diseases	
Systemic Arthritides	Systemic, multi-organ conditions which affect the temporomandibular joint, e.g. Rheumatoid arthritis, Lupus erythematosus
Condylosis/idiopathic condylar resorption	Idiopathic degenerative condition which results in loss of condylar height and progressive anterior open bite
Osteochondritis dissecans	TMJ pain and restricted mouth opening caused by cartilage and bony portions idiopathically breaking free within the joint space
Osteonecrosis	Death of bone within the TMJ complex
Joint neoplasm	Benign or malignant neoplastic growths within the TMJ complex. Examples include osteosarcoma, malignant ameloblastoma, squamous cell carcinoma
Synovial chondromatosis	Cartilaginous metaplasia of mesenchymal remnants of the synovial tissue of joint. The cartilaginous nodules form loose bodies within the joint space
Fractures	
Fracture	Fracture of any bone within the TMJ complex, most common being condylar fracture
Congenital/developmental disorders	
Aplasia	Absence of condyle and incomplete development of articular fossa and eminence, resulting in facial asymmetry
Hypoplasia	Incomplete or underdevelopment of condyle or fossa
Hyperplasia	Non-neoplastic over development of cranial bones. May affect condyle or entire mandible
Masticatory muscle disorders	
Tendonitis	Pain of tendon origin affected by jaw movement. Pain replicated by palpating tendon. Temporalis tendon is most commonly affected
Myositis	Pain of muscular origin with clinical characteristics of inflammation or infection, e.g. oedema, erythema, pyrexia
Spasm	Sudden, involuntary, reversible tonic contraction of a muscle
Muscular contracture	Shortening of muscle due to fibrosis of tendons, ligaments or muscle fibres
Muscular hypertrophy	Enlargement of one or more of masticatory muscles
Muscular neoplasm	Neoplasm of masticatory muscles which may be benign, malignant or metastatic, e.g. Myoma, rhabdomyosarcoma
Movement disorders	
Orofacial dyskinesia	Involuntary repetitive movements of the mouth and face, most common in older patients taking long-term anti-psychotic medications
Oromandibular dystonia	Rare motor disorder which results in focal dystonia (Involuntary, repetitive, sustained muscle contractions) which affects muscles of facial expression and muscles of mastication

(continued)

Table 4 (continued)

Condition	Description
Masticatory muscle pain attributed to systemic/central pain disorders	
Masticatory muscle pain attributed to systemic/central pain disorders	Chronic continuous muscle pain, aggravated by function, caused by systemic conditions, e.g. fibromyalgia, complex regional pain syndrome
Associated structures	
Coronoid hyperplasia	Progressive enlargement of coronoid process. This can result in impeded mandibular opening when obstructed by zygomatic process of maxilla

Based on information from Schiffman et al. [17]

References

1. Yanagi Y, Asaumi J, Maki Y, Murakami J, Hisatomi M, Matsuzaki H, Konouchi H, Honda Y, Kishi K. Incidentally found and unexpected tumors discovered by MRI examination for temporomandibular joint arthrosis. Eur J Radiol. 2003;47(1):6–9. https://doi.org/10.1016/s0720-048x(03)00095-0. PMID: 12810214.
2. Bullitt E, Tew JM, Boyd J. Intracranial tumors in patients with facial pain. J Neurosurg. 1986;64(6):865–71. https://doi.org/10.3171/jns.1986.64.6.0865. PMID: 3009737.
3. Beecroft E, et al. Management of painful Temporomandibular disorder in adults. NHS England Getting It Right First Time (GIRFT) and Royal College of Surgeons' Faculty of Dental Surgery; 2024; Available from: https://www.rcseng.ac.uk/dental-faculties/fds/publications-guidelines/clinical-guidelines/.
4. Crawford CE, Srinivas A, Momin P, Watts J, Davies SJ, Pemberton MN. Early identification of malignancy in trismus: ten-year evolution of a trismus checklist to improve patient safety. Br Dent J. 2022; https://doi.org/10.1038/s41415-022-4310-y.
5. Durham J, Ohrbach R, Baad-Hansen L, Davies S, De Laat A, Goncalves DG, Gordan VV, Goulet JP, Häggman-Henrikson B, Horton M, Koutris M, Law A, List T, Lobbezoo F, Michelotti A, Nixdorf DR, Oyarzo JF, Peck C, Penlington C, Raphael KG, Santiago V, Sharma S, Svensson P, Visscher CM, Yoshiki I, Alstergren P, INfORM. Constructing the brief diagnostic criteria for temporomandibular disorders (bDC/TMD) for field testing. J Oral Rehabil. 2024;51(5):785–94.
6. Petersson A. What you can and cannot see in TMJ imaging–an overview related to the RDC/TMD diagnostic system. J Oral Rehabil. 2010;37:771. Wiley Online Library.
7. Gray RJ, Quayle AA, Horner K. The effects of positioning variations in transcranial radiographs of the temporomandibular joint: a laboratory study. Br J Oral Maxillofac Surg. 1991;29(4):241–9.
8. Slade GD, Bair E, Greenspan JD, Dubner R, Fillingim RB, Diatchenko L, et al. Signs and symptoms of first-onset TMD and sociodemographic predictors of its development: the OPPERA prospective cohort study. J Pain. 2013;14(12 Suppl):T20–32.e1-3.
9. Beddis HP, Davies SJ, Budenberg A, Horner K, Pemberton MN. Temporomandibular disorders, trismus and malignancy: development of a checklist to improve patient safety. Br Dent J. 2014;217:351–5.
10. Mahan PE, Alling CC. Facial pain. 3rd ed. Philadelphia: Lea & Febiger; 1991;27, 35, p. 150–51.

11. Kvåle A, Ljunggren AE, Johnsen TB. Palpation of muscle and skin. Is this a reliable and valid procedure in assessment of patients with long-lasting musculoskeletal pain? Eur J Phys. 2009; https://doi.org/10.1080/14038190310016526.
12. Stockstill JW, Gross AJ, McCall WD Jr. Interrater reliability in masticatory muscle palpation. J Craniomandib Disord. 1989;3(3):143–6.
13. Beddis HP, Pemberton MN, Davies SJ. Sleep bruxism: an overview for clinicians. Br Dent J. 2018;225:497–502.
14. Durham J, Steele JG, Wassell RW, Exley C. Living with uncertainty: temporomandibular disorders. J Dent Res. 2010;89(8):827–30.
15. Schiffman E, Ohrbach R, Truelove E, Look J, Anderson G, Goulet JP, et al. Diagnostic Criteria for Temporomandibular Disorders (DC/TMD) for clinical and research applications: recommendations of the International RDC/TMD Consortium Network and Orofacial Pain Special Interest Group. J Oral Facial Pain Headache. 2014;28(1):6–27.
16. Beecroft E, et al. Temporomandibular disorder for the general dental practitioner. Prim Dent J. 2019;7(4):62–70.
17. Schiffman E, et al. Diagnostic Criteria for Temporomandibular Disorders (DC/TMD) for Clinical and Research Applications: recommendations of the International RDC/TMD Consortium Network* and Orofacial Pain Special Interest Group†. J Oral Facial Pain Headache. 2014;28(1):6–27.
18. van der Meer HA, Speksnijder CM, Engelbert RHH, Lobbezoo F, Nijhuis-van der Sanden MWG, Visscher CM. The association between headaches and temporomandibular disorders is confounded by bruxism and somatic symptoms. Clin J Pain. 2017;33(9):835–43.
19. Vivaldi D, Di Giosia M, Tchivileva IE, Jay GW, Slade GD, Lim PF. Headache attributed to TMD is associated with the presence of comorbid bodily pain: a case-control study. Headache. 2018;58(10):1593–600.
20. Réus JC, Polmann H, Souza BDM, Flores-Mir C, Gonçalves DAG, de Queiroz LP, et al. Association between primary headaches and temporomandibular disorders: a systematic review and meta-analysis. J Am Dent Assoc. 2022;153(2):120–31.e6.
21. Tchivileva IE, Ohrbach R, Fillingim RB, Lin F-C, Lim PF, Arbes SJ, et al. Clinical, psychological, and sensory characteristics associated with headache attributed to temporomandibular disorder in people with chronic myogenous temporomandibular disorder and primary headaches. J Headache Pain. 2021;22(1):42.

Psychological Considerations

Chris Penlington and Richard Ohrbach

In this chapter, we will discuss:

The importance of recognising pain as an *alarm,* which can be triggered not only by physical damage but also because the sensitivity of the alarm itself changes in different circumstances
Common psychological and social risk factors for pain becoming persistent, how to help and how to avoid making things worse
The concept of supported self-management
When to consider making a referral to specialist services

Often TMD have short-term symptoms that respond well to simple management. The focus of this chapter is specifically on the painful subtypes of TMD, which at times can result in persistent pain. A TMD might also, however, represent one element of a larger set of pain conditions that are not simply limited to the jaw and face.

It is critical that dental care professionals can recognise that acute pain (short-term, <3 months' duration) and persistent pain (≥3 months' duration) are very different. Both acute and persistent pain should be understood in terms of the biopsychosocial model [1], which means that biological, psychological and social factors affect all forms of pain to greater or lesser extents dependent on a variety of factors.

C. Penlington (✉)
School of Dental Sciences,, Newcastle University, Newcastle upon Tyne, UK
e-mail: chris.penlington@newcastle.ac.uk

R. Ohrbach
Oral Diagnostic Sciences, University at Buffalo, Buffalo, NY, USA
e-mail: ohrbach@buffalo.edu

S. Davies et al. (eds.), *Temporomandibular Disorders in Primary Dental Care*,
BDJ Clinician's Guides, https://doi.org/10.1007/978-3-032-01301-9_4

Acute pain is generally associated with observable biological factors underlying some form of actual or potential tissue damage—which dentists are most familiar with. Having said that, dentists are also aware of how situational anxiety or an anxious parent in the consulting room will affect acute pain.

In contrast, persistent pain, often without identifiable ongoing biological pathology, is strongly affected by psychological and social factors, and those factors should be incorporated into any management plans for persistent pain.

1 Can a GDP Understand Persistent Pain?

If persistent pain is an unfamiliar concept, it's worth taking time to understand it. Persistent pain is *different* to acute pain and requires *different management*. Risks of not recognising this include ineffective management strategies, loss of trust and iatrogenic harm. In the past, it has even been common for practitioners to stigmatise patients who continue to experience pain following treatment by blaming them or labelling their pain as "psychological", thus perpetuating distress. There are several factors that may make understanding about persistent pain challenging for general dental practitioners:

1. Pain studies do not feature to any significant extent in the dental under-graduate or post-graduate curricula or in training pathways. This means that the dental graduate has not had the advantage of thinking that pain might be anything other than a simple reaction or sensation to a noxious stimulus. Pain is rarely the product only of a noxious stimulus, and often in persistent pain, other factors become more significant than nociception in the perpetuation and worsening of pain.
2. The pain that dental patients experience is, in most cases, an acute pain, associated with inflammation and/or infection. These pain, such as pulpitis, follow a relatively simple cause-and-effect pattern. If the cause is addressed, the pain is usually short-lived. After the resolution of an acute pain episode, it is reasonable to expect that the patient will return to their previous status with no lasting consequences. It is entirely reasonable that repeated experiences of this nature will set the expectation in the mind of the dental clinician that pain always functions in this way.
3. The diagnosis of a persistent pain is much more complex than the diagnosis of an acute pain. It will usually require a considerable investment of time with the patient and is often a diagnosis of exclusion. For a dentist used to working within a clearly delineated model of cause and effect, it is likely to feel unfamiliar and uncomfortable, especially when working with patients who have similar expectations about pain.

Developing a comprehensive understanding of pain based on modern science is likely to be challenging and to take time, but is necessary, in order to provide optimal management to patients who experience persistent painful TMD or other orofacial pain conditions.

2 Pain

In chapter "Functional Anatomy and Pain Science", it is discussed that pain is an *alarm*. It is not an accurate indicator of physical damage, injury or tooth decay. Pain is generated *in the brain*, in response to nociceptive signals from the body and contextual cues from elsewhere in the brain. The brain processes these signals to determine if the response of pain is warranted and how much. There are two implications of this for dentists treating TMD:

1. Pain in the brain engenders further responses, and those responses are important. Any strong negative emotions or evaluations that are associated with the experience of pain become part of the information used by the brain in continuing to generate pain. The social context is equally important, signalling safety in situations where a person feels validated, respected and confident in their dentist or signalling danger if these conditions are not met.

   Neural activity underlying the pain system can therefore be influenced by the dentist's confidence in implementing a management plan that will allow the patient to feel understood and supported. The way in which you, as a dental care professional, listen to a patient, take their concerns seriously, give a careful explanation and share an appropriate management plan will play an important part in the prognosis. The importance of an early explanation of symptoms and of being validated were important findings in a study of the experiences of patients living with painful TMD [2].
2. Psychological and social factors in general (e.g. general life stressors) also feed into this system. They *do not cause* pain but have a strong role, which can intensify pain or make it more likely to persist. These factors therefore need careful management. It is particularly important that your explanations or interventions as a dental care professional do not add to any existing distress. For example, it is important that the explanations you give do not cause the patient to think that you do not believe their pain or to think you believe their pain is "in their head". It is essential when treating any type of TMD to emphasize from the beginning that the active engagement of the patient in following your recommendations is important. Active engagement in self-management strategies (see below) can be described as the foundation on which other management options will rest—on many occasions, these things *are* the management plan.

   It is important to recognise that often the *consequences* of pain can also *maintain or exacerbate* pain. This is essentially why self-management is so important. If we imagine that pain is like a burning fire, some of the impacts of pain, including mood, muscle tension and loss of sleep, become like additional fuel to the fire. Even in cases where we are not able to resolve the pain, minimising

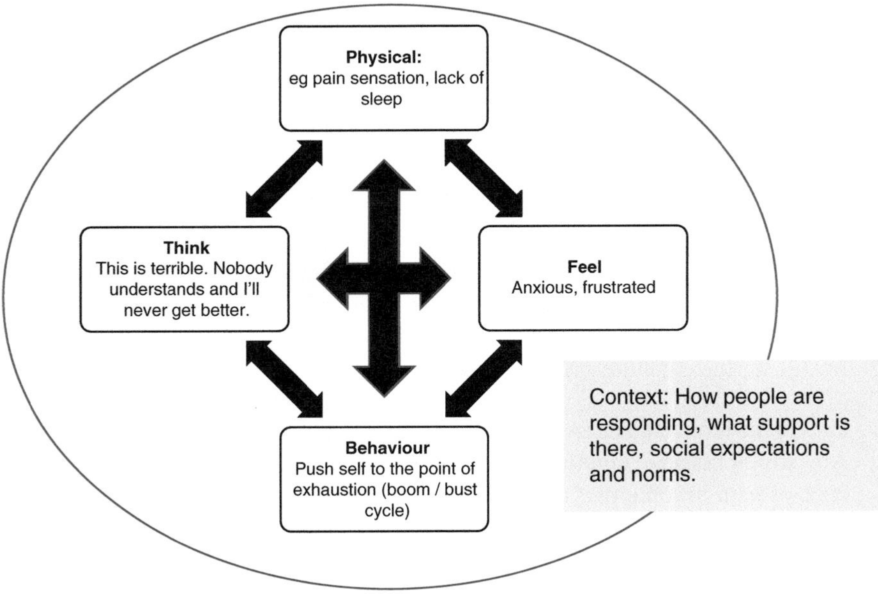

Fig. 1 A possible CBT formulation of how different elements of the experience may interrelate

these impacts is likely to be helpful. This is a basic application of cognitive behavioural therapy (CBT), also sometimes referred to as the five areas model. The premise of CBT is that because thoughts, emotions, physical sensations, behaviours and the environment are interrelated, small initial changes in one or more areas can lead to significant impacts overall. Figure 1 shows one possible way in which different aspects of the pain experience may be related, based on CBT.

3 Risk Factors

The two most important factors that have been associated with risk of TMD progressing into a persistent pain problem are intensity of pain and number of other painful conditions [3]. For patients with jaw pain complaints, it is important to ask about pain that they might experience in other areas of the body. A pain manikin can very rapidly and efficiently help screen for the number and extent of other pain problems.

Mental health conditions including anxiety and depression also commonly occur alongside TMD. Mental health conditions do not cause TMD or other pains, but such conditions can make symptoms more difficult to manage. It is important that any known mental health conditions are well managed. Patients should be advised to speak with their GP or a mental health professional if there are mental health concerns or conditions. Referral routes will differ between countries—in England, self-referral to Talking Therapies services is possible, and the relevant local service can be searched on the Internet.

Some psychological and social factors have specifically been linked to increased risk of pain becoming persistent and warrant special attention. The assessment of these factors can be easily remembered by the mnemonic FLATS [4]. Table 1 lists some quick ways of assessing each of these areas.

Any positive response in the FLATS assessment might indicate a higher risk of progression to or maintenance of persistent pain and therefore warrant increased importance of considering psychosocial factors with any established physical factors.

If patients respond positively to at least one of the above risk factors, they should be offered appointments at intervals of 3 months or less for monitoring, support and reinforcement of self-management recommendations. For patients with three or more of the above risk factors, or where disabling pain has persisted for 6 months or more, immediate referral to specialist treatment is recommended.

Recommendations for managing the above risk factors in primary care are shown in Table 2.

Table 1 FLATS acronym for identifying factors associated with increased risk of pain becoming persistent

Factor associated with increased risk of pain becoming persistent	Assess by use of validated instrument	Or assessed more simply by a single YES/NO question
Fear of pain	Tampa Scale of Kinesiophobia for TMD [5] somatic focus subscale	Do you worry that you could cause injury by biting, chewing or making certain jaw movements?
Low mood and anxiety	PHQ4 [6] 4 item scale	Do you often feel sad, depressed, nervous or worried?
Avoidance of functional movement	Tampa Scale of Kinesiophobia for TMD [5] activity avoidance scale	Do you avoid certain jaw movements because of pain?
Thinking the worst	Pain Catastrophizing Scale [7]	Do you have thoughts about your pain such as "it's terrible and it's never going to get any better"?
Social impact of pain	Family Impact of Pain Scale [8]	Are you concerned that your pain has an impact on other people?

Table 2 Suggestions for management in primary care in respect of common psychological and social risk factors

Factor associated with increased risk of pain becoming persistent	Notes on management of this factor
Fear of pain	This kind of fear often represents a belief or worry that: the pain is a symptom of a more serious condition; the cause of the pain has not been correctly diagnosed; or the pain will become so severe and long-lasting that it will overwhelm the person's capacity to cope. Long periods of uncertainty are unhelpful to patients and likely to increase fear, so it is recommended to make an early diagnosis, which can be provisional if confirmatory tests or specialist referrals are required. An adequate physical examination, a clear diagnosis, a comprehensive explanation and a management plan that incorporates attention to physical reassessment and clinician monitoring of the condition as well as self-efficacy will usually be helpful in alleviating this type of fear
Low mood and anxiety	Low mood or anxiety may be related to pain and its impact; they can also be related to other conditions or situations and thereby unrelated to the pain. If mood or anxiety problems have persisted, patients should be encouraged to self-refer for psychological therapy or speak to their GP
Avoidance of functional movement	For acute pain or on initial presentation, recommending a pain-free diet of soft food for up to 2 weeks minimizes unnecessary loading and strain and allows the jaw to rest. This allows for any inflammation to settle and avoids additional strain on sore muscles or joints. Any altered chewing patterns, such as avoidance of one side because of pain, should be corrected with bilateral chewing. After 2 weeks, patients should be encouraged to gradually return to normal use of the jaw Beyond 2 weeks, there is little additional benefit, and restriction can actually interfere with recovery in that restoration of normal function is part of pain rehabilitation. Continuing to avoid jaw movement beyond this time may be associated with fear of pain and beliefs that movement is exacerbating an underlying problem Give guidance to gradually increase the range of movement, and provide reassurance that this is not causing damage even if painful
Thinking the worst	Thinking the worst, or catastrophising, is a style of thinking that is common in response to pain. In the first instance, it is important to communicate clinical information clearly (see fear of pain in row 2). Having done this, if a patient expresses "worst-case-scenario" thinking, you can remind them of clinical information previously discussed. It may also be helpful to reassure patients that it's natural to think the worst about pain but that this doesn't mean that the thoughts are likely to be true. Encourage patients to focus on positive interests and give less attention to this type of thinking and to pain
Social impact of pain	Concerns about being a burden or not able to fulfil responsibilities are common and make it difficult for patients to focus on looking after their own needs. Encourage communication with family and friends about reasonable adjustments to plans while pain remains troublesome. Family and friends often want to help but don't know how to or what they should suggest. Consider providing information for family and friends as well as information targeted to the patient themselves

4 Supported Self-Management

Supported self-management of all subtypes of TMD is recommended as a first-line treatment by the Royal College of Surgeons of England [9] and the American Association for Dental Research [10]. Guidelines for self-management can be found in chapter "Management". If pain becomes persistent, patients will benefit from also accessing additional self-management support and from developing their own plan to develop or maintain a broader range of healthy habits and minimise the impact of pain on their life. As pain persists, the prospect of complete resolution becomes less likely, and effective self-management becomes the primary management strategy.

Practitioners may suggest to their patients that as their condition is multi-faceted, it will require a multidisciplinary team—and that the patient is an essential member of that team! Self-management refers to actions that a patient can do themselves to minimise their pain and its impact on their life. Even if pain does not resolve completely, many patients are able to use regular self-management strategies that keep their pain under control and limit the impact that it has on their life. Self-management support refers to what health professionals do to help patients with self-management. In the dental practice, this includes giving accurate, good-quality information and recommendations. Where possible, recommendations should be reinforced with provision of written information.

Signposting to additional resources for self-management of pain may also be helpful.

Figure 2 shows an example of a pain cycle available on livewellwithpain.co.uk, one example of an online resource which patients can use to guide their attention to

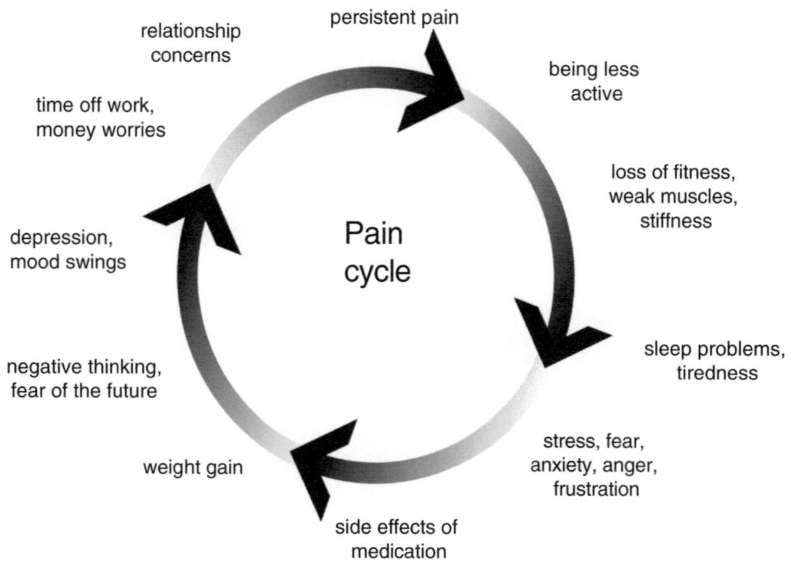

Fig. 2 Illustration of a pain cycle

a broad range of changeable issues that they can work on to impact their pain over time.

An adapted version specific to TMD is shown below. Many of the ways in which TMD impact everyday life become problems in their own right and can serve as maintaining and exacerbating factors for continued pain. Patients who are able to recognise that this may have relevance to their experience of pain can be signposted to self-management support resources for help in addressing some of these ongoing impacts (Fig. 3).

The self-care cycle illustrates the range of activities that can be cultivated and are likely to be helpful for the self-management of pain that has become persistent. It is helpful for dental team members to be aware of the wide range of potential impacts of pain that becomes persistent and that a wide range of strategies may therefore be required. It is useful to become aware of local resources that are available to support self-management of pain and to be able to signpost to relevant national and international resources.

Figure 4 shows skills, strategies and attributes that are helpful for the self-management of persistent pain. Introduction of these skills may occur in any order depending on individual factors and preferences; the key is that many different factors and a range of different strategies and approaches are likely to be relevant to the self-management of pain that has become persistent.

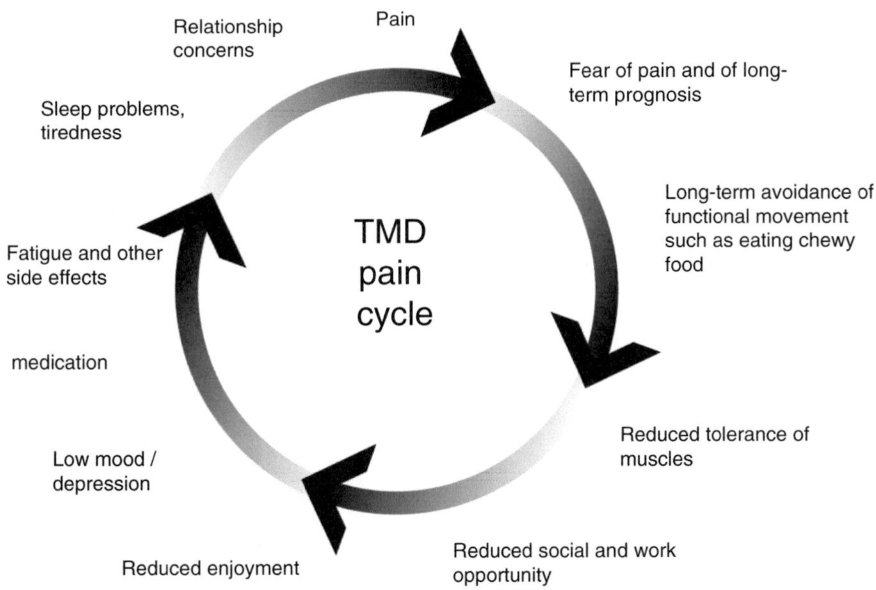

Fig. 3 Pain cycle for TMD. (Adapted with permission from Livewellwithpain.co.uk pain cycle)

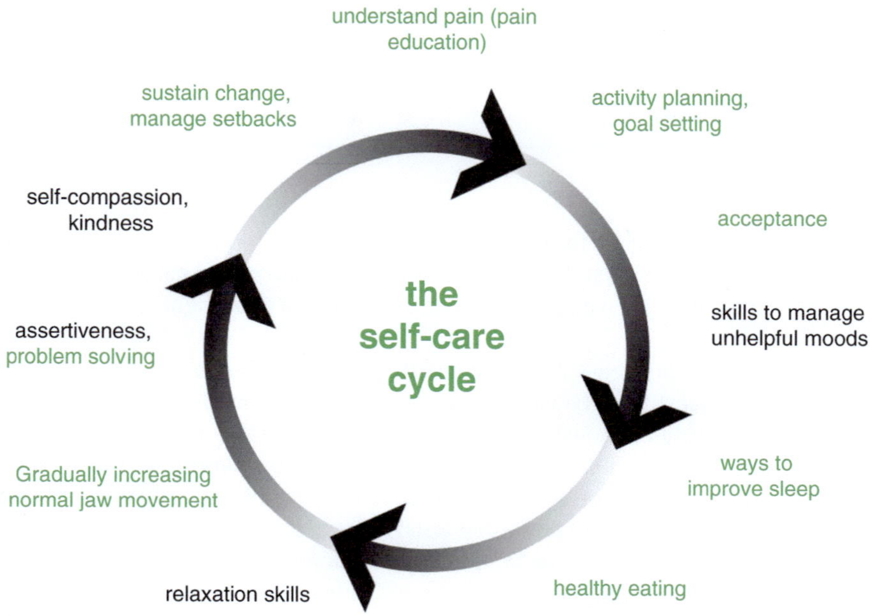

Fig. 4 Self-care cycle for the self-management of persistent pain

5 Sleep

Sleep is frequently disturbed in pain conditions; poor sleep often contributes to the onset of persistent pain conditions and to the persistence of pain. Whereas an acute pain of, for example, toothache may disturb sleep due to its intensity, the impact of persistent pain on sleep is different. A wide range of factors may be important, including thoughts, feelings of anxiety, frustration and distress and habits. Although pain will always present a challenge to the ability to sleep, the poor sleep associated with persistent pain can often be improved with the right intervention. It is important to ask about sleep and to be able to give recommendations for improving sleep.

In childhood, people often have clear routines around sleep—a fixed bedtime, a routine to wind down before bed, calming environment or rules about not using electronic devices in bed. These simple strategies are known as "sleep hygiene", and they point to the structure whereby good sleep is a learned behaviour. If experiencing any difficulty with sleep, the first thing to do is to resume these healthy routines—any of us who have been around children at bedtime know that they are there for a reason! Patients can be guided to many online resources for information about how they can implement behaviours that will help improve their sleep; for example, Sleep - Live Well with Pain.

For some people, improving sleep hygiene on its own is not enough. Cognitive behaviour therapy for sleep (CBT-sleep) is highly effective, and apps such as

Sleepio, Sleepstation or Pzizz can also be helpful. In some countries, these are available through prescription, so patients should speak with their GP about the different options available.

6 Reassurance

It is natural that pain leads to worry, especially when the pain is intense. At initial consultation, it is important that all necessary investigations are carried out, and a thorough explanation is given to the patient. This is likely to be highly reassuring for the patient.

Some patients may request further investigations at subsequent visits, and the basis for that request must be carefully considered. For example, new information regarding previously unknown symptom patterns indicative of potential pathology would be a reasonable indication for further investigation. Worry, by itself, and a need for further reassurance is not an indication for further investigation. In that instance, it is important to not do further tests: any reassurance gained from an additional negative test result will be temporary. Additional testing must be contrasted with the possibility that any test can identify possible deviations from ideal anatomy that may be completely normal and unrelated to the clinical complaints—but which can serve as an additional source of worry. A negative investigation is also likely to feed into a cycle of increasing worry over time, since the patient will likely come to doubt that particular investigation.

Frequent reassurance-seeking itself can increase worry or anxiety through a process of *negative reinforcement*. Repeated reassurance can temporarily reduce worry, and therefore, seeking reassurance can become strongly reinforced as a pattern of behaviour. Patients who repeatedly and excessively request reassurance should be gently reminded of previous findings and encouraged to remind themselves what was discussed previously. If the issue persists, consider signposting to psychological services for management of anxiety.

7 "There's nothing wrong"

Words matter. The message that "there is nothing wrong" in the presence of pain is unhelpful and likely to cause worry, distress and feelings of being misunderstood. Instead, describe findings in detail, including what has been investigated and the results of these investigations. Explain that pain can be an alarm, that this is a real and well-known mechanism of pain and that different management strategies are needed for this kind of pain. Explain that pain can persist after its original cause has resolved and that the presence of pain is then a false alarm, affected by many other factors. Suggest that it is important to work on as many of these factors as possible. Signpost to self-management resources, or refer to your local pain clinic. Be sure to acknowledge the experience of pain regardless of whether you can find pathology that would usually account for it.

8 Onward Referral

For patients whose needs exceed those that can be managed in routine practice, referral to psychological services or a pain clinic may be indicated.

Consider advising patients to self-refer to psychological services if the patient acknowledges that anxiety or depression is impacting on overall functioning or may be contributing to their ability to manage their pain. Similarly recommend that patients seek a referral to psychology services if they disclose that past emotionally traumatic experiences are having an impact. Patients may be able to access a range of psychological therapies including CBT (cognitive behavioural therapy), EMDR (eye-movement desensitization and reprocessing), ACT (acceptance and commitment therapy), systemic therapy, CFT (compassion-focused therapy) or counselling. Likewise, patients may benefit from mindfulness, health coaching or social prescribing if they are able to access these services in their area.

For patients who are less clear about the impact of psychological factors or for whom the experience of pain is the overwhelming problem, consider referring to a pain clinic. Pain clinics are staffed by multidisciplinary teams of staff often representing psychology, physiotherapy, occupational therapy and medicine who can work together to address a range of issues that may be having an impact on the pain and its severity.

Regardless of whether you make an onward referral, regular routine follow-up is important to continue to provide grounded reassurance that the initial complaint of pain is being taken seriously and that any change in the symptom severity will be appropriately and timely noted. In the absence of such symptom worsening, the dentist should continue to follow the guidelines outlined in the chapter.

In this chapter, we have learned that:

Psychological and social factors, both before and after the onset of a persistent pain, can influence pain and its prognosis but do not cause pain
There are some simple ideas for management of common psychological and social factors in the surgery
Supporting self-management, or the things that a patient does themselves to manage their pain and its impact, is a critical part of management of TMD
There are some reasons for making onward referral to specialist psychology or pain services

References

1. Ohrbach R. Biopsychosocial aspects of orofacial pain. In: Farah CS, editor. Contemporary oral medicine. Heidelberg: Springer Meteor; 2018. p. 1–21.
2. Durham J, Steele JG, Wassell RW, Exley C. Living with uncertainty: temporomandibular disorders. J Dent Res. 2010;89(8):827–30.

3. Slade GD, Ohrbach R, Greenspan JD, Fillingim RB, Bair E, Sanders AE, et al. Painful temporomandibular disorder: decade of discovery from OPPERA studies. J Dent Res. 2016;95(10):1084–92.
4. Beecroft E, Penlington C, Desai H, Durham J. Temporomandibular disorder for the general dental practitioner. Prim Dent J. 2019 Feb;19(7):62–70.
5. Visscher CM, Ohrbach R, van Wijk AJ, Wilkosz M, Naeije M. The Tampa Scale for Kinesiophobia for temporomandibular disorders (TSK-TMD). Pain. 2010;150(3):492–500.
6. Löwe B, Wahl I, Rose M, Spitzer C, Glaesmer H, Wingenfeld K, et al. A 4-item measure of depression and anxiety: validation and standardization of the Patient Health Questionnaire-4 (PHQ-4) in the general population. J Affect Disord. 2010;122(1):86–95.
7. Sullivan MJL, Bishop SR, Pivik J. The pain catastrophizing scale: development and validation. Psychol Assess. 1995;7(4):524–32.
8. Newton-John TR. The family impact of pain scale: preliminary validation. J Clin Psychol Med Settings. 2005;12(4):349–58.
9. Durham J. Summary of Royal College of Surgeons' (England) clinical guidelines on management of temporomandibular disorders in primary care. Br Dent J. 2015;218(6):355–6.
10. Greene CS. Managing the care of patients with temporomandibular disorders. J Am Dent Assoc. 2010;141(9):1086–8.

Management of Temporomandibular Disorders

Emma Beecroft, Chris Penlington, and Justin Durham

1 Introduction

The complexity of temporomandibular disorders (TMD) can feel overwhelming for clinicians; management however does not have to be. This chapter aims to outline the main strategies for management for TMD. Each treatment plan will be individual to the patient, but there are essential foundations of TMD management, which should be consistent for all TMD cases, whether acute or persistent in nature. Additional tailored interventions can be added for patients; however, the essential foundations of TMD management support the patient in the longer-term and will help improve prognosis.

2 Essential Foundations for TMD Management

I. *Biopsychosocial Approach*

Biological, psychological, and social management elements should be delivered through a single integrated treatment plan. The biopsychosocial approach is explored further in Chapter "Psychological Considerations".

E. Beecroft (✉) · C. Penlington · J. Durham
School of Dental Sciences, Newcastle University, Newcastle upon Tyne, UK
e-mail: emma.beecroft@newcastle.ac.uk; chris.penlington@newcastle.ac.uk; justin.durham@newcastle.ac.uk

S. Davies et al. (eds.), *Temporomandibular Disorders in Primary Dental Care*, BDJ Clinician's Guides, https://doi.org/10.1007/978-3-032-01301-9_5

II. *Education and Reassurance*

Education and reassurance; empower the patient; facilitate understanding of the condition for the individual and their family, friends, and work colleagues; perpetuate active engagement with ongoing management in order to improve outcome.

III. *Supported Self-Management*

Supported self-management are a group of interventions recommended by the clinician at initial point of diagnosis, which when completed by the patient are highly likely to have positive therapeutic effect.

IV. *Reversible and Non-invasive*

As 75–90% of TMD patients respond to conservative treatment strategies, initial management should be reversible and non-invasive.

V. *Engagement*

If an individual living with TMD does not positively engage with their care, progress is likely to be challenging. Clinicians must facilitate and maintain engagement through the course of the individual's condition and highlight the need to work in a therapeutic partnership.

3 Education and Reassurance

Time should be spent to explain about TMD and discuss its aetiology and pathogenesis in a manner a lay person can understand. A clear individual diagnosis should be provided for the patient, explaining the diagnosis in relation to the symptoms the individual is feeling will help them take ownership of their condition, Box 1 provides support on how to phrase such discussions (Box 1).

For persistent TMD, education at the point of diagnosis should include a discussion about the role of psychological factors including anxiety, depression, and thinking the worst. As explained in Chapter "Psychological Considerations", these *do not cause* pain but are known to contribute to the intensity and maintenance of pain once it is present and are likely themselves to be triggered by pain. Introducing the relationship between psychosocial factors and the individual's pain at an early stage will promote understanding and engagement with the full remit of management strategies. Dental clinicians traditionally find such discussions difficult. Box 2 aims to show how these discussions can be managed empathetically by providing some examples of how these conversations can be had.

Positive reassurance should focus on the benign and largely non-progressive nature of TMD. Naeije et al. found disc displacement to be highly prevalent;

Box 1 Examples of lay terminology which could be used to explain TMD aetiology and pathogenesis to patients

Reassurance as to the benign nature of TMD

"With TMD, the pain that you feel does not indicate that there is damage occurring within the jaw joint or the structures surrounding it. Continuing to use your jaw normally will not make the condition worse".

Explanation of persistent myogenous TMD

"With your condition, the main muscles which move the jaw are sending pain signals when they should not be because there is no actual injury within the muscle. The nerves within these muscles are hyper-responsive. Imagine them as a stereo and their volume switch turned to maximum. They are sending very loud, very **real** pain signals to highlight these muscles to you in a bid to protect them. It is your body working in an over-protective nature, meaning you are feeling significant pain when the muscle has no injury".

Explanation of disc displacement with reduction

"The lower jaw sits within a bony curve in the skull. Between the lower jaw and the skull lies a disc of cartilage which acts as a cushion allowing smooth movement when the jaw opens and closes. In some people, the disc moves further one way or another during opening or closing. The click that you hear is the disc moving back in to position between the lower jaw and the skull. Approximately 30% of all adults have a "clicky jaw". The click itself is normal for your jaw joint. The click does not mean there is any damage taking place to the disc or the jaw joint. We now understand that overtime the disc remodels. For some people, this means a click may start or stop. The aim of management is to reduce the pain you feel and not to eliminate your click".

Explanation to manage expectations for likely course for persistent TMD:

"There is no one treatment which will eliminate all of the pain associated with TMD. There are lots of treatment strategies which will support pain management but cannot be guaranteed to eliminate pain. For people who have TMD, they will likely have symptoms to one degree or another throughout life. Symptoms will usually come in cycles with periods of no or significantly less pain followed by short periods of flare-up. Management strategies we can utilise will help reduce how often you feel pain and how severe the pain is when it is present".

18–35% of asymptomatic adults demonstrate disc displacement; the percentage of individual joints with a disc displacement ranged from 9% to 45%. Seventy-one to eighty percent of those with disc displacement with reduction remained stable, and only 10–30% of disc displacements progress to disc displacement without reduction. Fortunately, loss of reduction is rarely accompanied by symptoms of pain and limited mouth opening. For those with symptomatic disc displacement without

Box 2 Introduction of concept of psychosocial pain factors

Clinician: "Whilst we know that mood or anxiety does not cause TMD, we know that when they present, they can affect the success of the other types of treatment dentists can provide. So, to get more bang for our buck, it is important to manage these at the same time as providing management from the dental side of things".

Clinician: "Being in constant pain is wearing and draining on emotional resilience. Have you ever noticed your pain is worse when you are tired, stressed, run-down, or feeling low? Considering such factors as part of our management plan has been shown to reduce the intensity of pain in individuals with TMD".

Clinician: "I bet you do not feel like the person that you were before all this started. It is important to realise this. Taking time every day to engage in an activity which gives you joy, like seeing friends and socialising, can help you manage the effect your condition has on who you are".

Clinician: "We understand so much more about pain than we ever have. If every individual in this room had an identical injury, e.g. stubbed their toe, we would all feel a totally different pain. If I was having a difficult day, perhaps I slept poorly, perhaps I was having a stressful time at work, or my mood was low due to a difficult family situation, the pain I felt would be more severe as my body tries to protect me more aggressively in times of need. Managing the factors which influence how we feel pain will reduce the intensity of the pain we feel".

Clinician: "When we are stressed or low, emotions are amplified, and our fuse may be shorter with our partners. A situation which would not usually make us cry such as being late for work may make us burst into tears. TMD pain can be equally amplified and intensity levels increased in such situations. Taking positive steps to manage our stress and mood has been shown to reduce pain intensity in TMD".

reduction, signs and symptoms have a tendency to resolve, confirming a favourable natural course of disc displacement without reduction. Schiffman et al.'s work corroborated the positive natural course for arthrogenous TMDs. Over an 8-year period, 76% of disc displacements remained stable, 10% reversed, and 14% progressed. For degenerative joint disease, 71% remained stable, 14% reversed, and 15% progressed. Reassurance is a powerful management tool that should not be underestimated. Failure to provide adequate reassurance can lead to increased anxiety and exacerbation of symptom severity. In addition to education with regard to the condition generally, education as to tailored appropriate and time-limited analgesic use should be provided. This will be discussed later in this chapter.

4 Engagement

At the point of first diagnosis, ensuring patients understand that outcome of treatment is related more to what they do themselves with supportive self-management rather than treatment received passively from medical professionals should be clearly outlined to ensure active patient engagement.

Maintenance of engagement over time can be more difficult. Clinicians must understand that the persistent nature of TMD and lack of "cure" can be draining and motivation for self-management can wane, leading to the worsening of symptoms. It is important to acknowledge these and support patient engagement longitudinally. The power of a few quick, simple questions assessing current TMD symptoms, offering suggestions for continuation or adaptation of self-management strategies, alongside both ongoing reassurance with regard to benign nature of TMD, and positive motivation to re-engage should not be under-estimated.

It is important for individuals under the care of a specialist team for their TMD, that primary care practitioners continue to offer advice and deliver care within their remit alongside specialist intervention. Consistent, positive, cross specialism reinforcement supports engagement and offers the best prognostic opportunity for patients.

5 Holistic Management Considerations for TMD

There are a number of holistic management considerations which offer benefit for all individuals with TMD.

6 Clinician-Patient Relationship

The importance of clinician-patient interaction is poorly conceptualised by clinicians, yet successful TMD management hinges on this relationship. Patients need to feel that they are heard. The utilisation of the communication techniques listed in Table 1 can help clinicians forge a positive relationship from first consultation. It has been shown that empathetic positive communication in the healthcare setting can actually reduce pain.

When used well, the communication techniques in Table 1 provide important validation of the patient's experience and build a relationship of trust and partnership between the clinician and patient.

One additional feature required for positive clinician-patient relationship is the belief by the patient that their treatment provider is competent and knowledgeable to treat their condition. Time is the cornerstone of this. The patient must feel that their clinician has taken the time to complete a thorough clinical examination (as per Chapter "Examination and Diagnosis of Temporomandibular Disorders") and

Table 1 Positive communication techniques for patient consultation

Technique	Description
Active listening	Active listening is an essential component of productive discussion and serves the dual purpose of helping the clinician listen carefully and indicating to the patient that they are being listened to and thus taken seriously. It can be demonstrated to the patient through a wide range of verbal and non-verbal triggers; e.g. requesting clarification of salient points demonstrates to the patient they are being heard and that the clinical wants to understand correctly what they are trying to say. Utilisation of a combination of the techniques in this table will help the clinician display that they are actively listening to the patients
Signalling	Signalling is important for giving patients confidence that they are being listened to Examples of non-verbal signalling: Gestures such as putting down instruments demonstrates focus Maintaining eye contact confers interest Moderating body position and posture presents openness and acceptance Examples of verbal signalling: Encouragement and/or complementary statements can provide confidence to continue Appropriate questioning demonstrates engagement
Mirroring	Involves the clinician subtly mimicking the patient's body language, tone of voice, posture, gestures, or wording. Mirroring suggests cohesion and develops trust and rapport For example, if a patient is describing something sad, their tone of voice may become lower and their speech slightly slower. If a clinician responds to this with an upbeat, high pitch, this acts in conflict to the patients' mannerisms and suggests lack of understanding or empathy. The clinician mirroring the patient's speech pattern presents synchrony and is more positively received
Reflecting	Reflection involves repeating back to patients in some way what they have said. It strengthens the message that you are listening to them, is encouraging, allows for clarification of what they are saying, and may offer them new insights about what they are saying. Reflection can occur at a range of different levels *Simple reflection* involves simply repeating back to the patient a few of their own words and can be used to encourage them to carry on talking For example: *Patient*: "I worry about damaging my joint more if I eat the wrong sort of food" *Clinician*: "You worry that you will damage the joint because…" *Paraphrasing* involves the clinician relaying back to the patient the clinicians understanding of what the patient said as a question For example: *Patient*: "I know the splint is helping, but the pain in my jaw is so intense I need something else" *Clinician*: "What I am hearing is that you would like to explore other management options in addition to your splint?" *Verbalisation* is attempting to put into words what the patient has not been able to For example: *Patient*: "I don't know if I should start the amitriptyline for my jaw pain" *Clinician*: "Because you're concerned about the side effects?" Simple reflections, paraphrasing, and verbalising suggest acceptance and understanding and promote partnership between the clinician and patient

(continued)

Table 1 (continued)

Technique	Description
Summarising	Summarising what the patient has said back to them in their own words can demonstrate to the patient that they have been heard and that the clinician is believing their account and taking their concerns seriously
Empathy	Being able to communicate to the patient that you understand how they are feeling builds trust, reduces anxiety, and can be directly therapeutic. Using all the techniques in this table can help display empathy Empathetic communication can be shown by the clinician by responding to the patient with understanding and keeping the focus on the patient For example: *Clinician*: "From what you're telling me, your jaw pain is making talking at work really hard for you" *Clinician*: "I am sorry your jaw pain is so severe at the moment"

clearly described their diagnosis and pathogenesis. This will provide this confidence. The ability of the patient to engage fully with treatment suggestions will rest on the quality of, and their confidence in, the relationship with their clinician and is crucial particularly to successful patient engagement in self-management.

7 Expectation Management

Early management of patient expectations with regard to persistent TMD is crucial. As with all persistent pain conditions, a "cure" is unlikely. A more realistic expectation is that optimisation of supported self-management strategies can protect against functional limitation and reduce the impact of the patient's pain. Without this understanding, patients can become entrenched in a cycle of disappointment, frustration, and anxiety, which will both undermine the relationship with the clinician and adversely affect outcome.

8 Psychological Factors

Chapter "Psychological Considerations" offered information with regard to appropriate assessment of an individual's psychosocial status and management with regard to this aspect of their TMD condition. For individuals living with TMD, open discussion at first point of contact, explaining the interaction between pain maintenance and intensity, emotions, and psychological factors, supports acceptance. Delaying this explanation till much later into management can lead individuals to draw conclusion that their clinician believed the pain is "in their head", affecting trust and reducing the likelihood of positive engagement in psychosocial management strategies which have been shown to improve patient-related outcome measures across persistent pain conditions.

Box 3 Diaphragmatic breathing exercise

- Lie down on a flat surface; the head, neck and spine should be in line.
- Pillows can be used under the head and knees to increase comfort if required.
- Relax the shoulders.
- Place one hand on the middle of the chest; place the other hand on the stomach below the ribcage.
- Focus on your breathing.
- Slowly inhale through the nose. The stomach should raise first, pushing upwards against your hand. The chest should remain still.
- To exhale, let the stomach fall downwards whilst exhaling through pursed lips. Again, the chest should remain still.
- Continue inhaling and exhaling slowly and steadily in this manner.
- Complete for 5 min per day three times daily.
- The exercise can be completed seated or standing when individuals are comfortable with the technique.

Discussions can be complex, and so signposting patients to high-quality online resources such as "live well with pain" at https://my.livewellwithpain.co.uk/ supports patient interaction throughout the consultation period. All individuals living with TMD regardless of severity of psychosocial profile would benefit from a treatment plan with simple psychosocial strategies which decrease the impact of pain, such as taking time to do something they enjoy every day even if they are in pain or having a 30-minute walk in the fresh air once a day. Other beneficial techniques include advising patients to utilise diaphragmatic breathing, outlined in Box 3, which has been shown to facilitate relaxation, ease muscular tension, reduce pain, lower blood pressure and heart rate, lower cortisol (stress hormone) levels, manage anxiety, and improve both lung and cognitive functions.

9 Sleep Hygiene

Chapter "Psychological Considerations" explained psychosocially why sleep can be problematic in the presence of pain. From a biological perspective, persistent pain and sleep have a reciprocal relationship. Persistent pain is associated with poor sleep quality, presenting as issues with both initiation and maintenance of sleep. Poor sleep quality lowers pain tolerance and causes pain amplification. All individuals with persistent TMD would benefit from direction to simple sleep hygiene recommendations, highlighted in Box 4 to utilise at home to improve quality and quantity of sleep and in turn build resilience. The How to Sleep Well with Pain leaflet developed by the Live well with Pain team is available from https://livewellwithpain.co.uk/resources-for-people-with-pain/download-leaflets/ and is a positive resource, in addition to the app resources discussed in Chapter "Psychological Considerations".

Box 4 Simple sleep hygiene tips

- Create a sleep routine: Wake up and go to sleep at the same time each day.
- Reduce caffeine consumption throughout the day.
- Get adequate sunlight in the morning and throughout the day.
- Exercise in the morning, not evening.
- Avoid alcohol, sugar, and fatty foods in the evening.
- Avoid electronic devices in the hour before bedtime.
- Sleep in a dark, quiet, cool (15–19 degrees centigrade) environment.

10 Smoking Cessation

The incidence of TMD is higher in smokers than non-smokers. Nicotine affects pain perception; chronic exposure is associated with hyperalgesia. Smokers also demonstrate higher levels of anxiety, depression, and perceived stress, thus worsening psychosocial profile. Smoking cessation supports both persistent pain management and general health and should be encouraged for all individuals with TMD.

11 Excessive Caffeine

Persistent pain conditions are negatively impacted by excessive caffeine consumption. Caffeine increases the perception of pain through catecholamine release, sensitising muscle nociceptors. Patients with persistent pain should be advised to keep the intake of caffeine low. The equivalent of one strong (filter coffee or equivalent) cup of caffeinated coffee per day is a sensible and easily understandable metric to use, as well as suggesting switching to decaffeinated alternative beverages wherever possible.

12 Supported Self-Management (SSM)

What the patient does at home is more likely to have beneficial effect on their condition that what we, as clinicians, are able to complete chairside. SSM empowers patients to take an active role in managing their condition.

Internationally advised key components of SSM include:

- Education (which we have covered above)
- Self-exercise therapy
- Thermal modalities (heat and cold application)
- Self-massage techniques
- Dietary guidance to ensure adequate nutritional intake and continued functional use of the temporomandibular joint complex
- Addressing parafunctional habits such as clenching or nail biting

These interventions are practical, low-cost, and evidence informed, offering individuals tools to reduce pain, improve function, and regain confidence in using the jaw. The importance of SSM lies not only in its ability to reduce pain and disability but also in its promotion of psychological wellbeing and long-term health behaviours. By helping patients identify and manage lifestyle factors such as sleep, mood, activity levels, and relationships, SSM encourages a holistic approach to persistent pain.

13 Self-Exercise Therapy

Therapeutic jaw exercises for TMD are designed to enhance coordination, muscular control, and joint mobility. Foundational coordination exercises which would be expected to support all TMD include the "n-stretch", which promotes jaw retrusion through tongue placement to the hard palate, and mirror-guided straight opening to correct lateral deviation of mandibular opening, should it be present. For individuals with any myogenous TMD, isometric exercises target muscle function through the application of gentle resistance (placement of the hand to gently resist movement) during opening and lateral excursive jaw movements.

For restricted mouth opening due to either myofascial guarding or disc displacement with reduction with limited opening, static stretching can improve range of mandibular opening by gently sustaining mild tension at point of resistance. The application of covered ice over the temporomandibular joint lateral poles immediately before exercise and/or use of over-the-counter analgesics 1 hour prior to isometric stretching exercise can improve patient comfort, which has been shown to gradually improve range of mandibular opening when completed regularly. It must be ensured that gentle pressure is evenly applied so both the right and left muscles of mastication and temporomandibular joint complex are loaded equally when completing this exercise. Finally, for cases of disc displacement without reduction, controlled lateral movements whilst biting on a cotton roll to support tooth disclusion can aid in joint mobilisation.

14 Thermal Modalities

Applying moist heat or covered ice to painful muscles can help modulate pain signals and improve function by promoting blood flow (heat), reducing inflammation (ice), decreasing muscle tension (heat and ice), and increasing local pain threshold (heat and ice), all of which are supported by evidence for short-term relief of TMD pain.

Some people find heat most beneficial; others ice. Trialling 3 days of each to determine the most effective response for the individual is a sensible suggestion to offer patients. Patients should be encouraged to apply their chosen thermal modality for 15–20 min twice a day for at least 1 month to allow time for improvement, with longitudinal use as part of their normal self-care practice being the most effective way to generate positive results.

15 Self-Massage Techniques

Gentle massage of temporalis and masseter helps reduce myofascial tension, improve local blood circulation, and decrease muscle tenderness associated with TMD. Regular myofascial release may also enhance jaw mobility, reduce clenching habits, and support relaxation of overactive facial muscles, contributing to overall symptom reduction when integrated into daily care routine.

Patients should be shown how to isolate the masseter muscle between their index finger and thumb and advised to apply gentle pressure whilst massaging from top to bottom of the muscle five times and then back to the front of the muscle five times. For temporalis, gentle pressure should be applied to the muscle using the index and middle finger and circular movements to trace the size of a pound coin made in any area of the muscle which is tender. Massage should take no longer than 1 min for each muscle twice per day.

The Royal College of Surgeons, Faculty of Dental Surgery, and NHS England 2024 guideline for management of painful TMD in adults provides links to video resources accessible for both patients and clinicians to guide them through all supported self-management strategies. Dental clinicians should review and adapt the supported self-management plan to ensure that management remains aligned with the patient's needs over time.

16 Active Intervention

16.1 Splint Therapy

Absolute certainty as to both the mechanism of action and the effect of splint therapy is currently under question. Recent high-profile publications have concluded that when compared to physiotherapy, behavioural therapy, pharmacotherapy, counselling, and no treatment, there was no evidence of splints improving pain or mouth opening in patients with persistent TMD. Evidence shows potential benefit of full coverage splints in the management of myogenous TMDs and strong evidence for positive reduction of headache features in cases of headache attributed to TMD and individuals with any TMD and a concomitant primary headache disorder.

Splints are usually worn through the night to protect the dentition from parafunction and provide an element of biofeedback to the patient. The term "malocclusion" [literally "bad bite"] suggests an occlusion can be wrong. This does not stand up to the observation that all dentists will have made: many of our patients have what we might consider a difficult occlusion which are far removed from what we might consider as normal. Yet the vast majority of these patients have no adverse reaction to these occlusions. That is why several authors, referenced elsewhere in this book, have argued that a better term is "maladaptive occlusion". Now we are judging an occlusion, not against a set of arbitrary rules or preconceptions but against the adaptive capability of that patient, at that time in their life. Surely, this elevates us from being oral engineers to being oral physicians. This has relevance when considering splint therapy. It is better to consider that a contribution that a splint can make to the reduction of a patient's symptoms is more due to relief from their existing occlusion than the provision of any occlusal pattern. Think of a splint as an occlusal holiday; it is not the template for what the patient needs. A course of successful splint therapy can have benefits well beyond its period of use [nobody needs to be on holiday forever].

Splints can be worn on upper or lower arches, and there is no evidence for improved efficacy for one over the other. The splint should be provided on the arch which has the largest number of teeth, but you can be guided by patient preference. Soft polyethylene soft splints (soft splints) or acrylic hard splints (stabilisation splints) can be used. There is no evidence for increased success in the literature between soft or hard splints, and therefore GDPs should provide a splint they feel comfortable designing, fitting, and maintaining. Subjectively, the authors of this chapter who work in specialist orofacial pain settings report increased success in terms of patient compliance, pain reduction, and functional improvement from hard acrylic stabilisation splints, but the patient cohort treated by these clinicians is likely to represent more refractory persistent TMD cases less representative of the TMD population as a whole.

Splints should be full coverage to protect from unfavourable dento-alveolar compensation and should not be provided to individuals with active dental disease (decay, unstable periodontal condition, poor oral hygiene) as risk of progression of dental disease will outweigh potential benefits.

Once provided, splints should be monitored by GDPs to ensure positive fit and even occlusal contacts in inter-cuspal position, and replacement should be arranged for evidence of excessive wear or damage. There is strong evidence for efficacy of splints over the short term. Long-term use for periods of greater than 6 months has not been shown to be beneficial, and therefore, once a patient's TMD has stabilised, continued use of the appliance is not essential; the splint can be reintroduced for short periods at times of cyclical flare-up.

Splints will have no effect on TMJ noises (click) in arthrogenous TMDs, and therefore, splint therapy for an asymptomatic disc displacement is not justifiable. The use of anterior repositioning splints to recapture disc position was historically popular. New evidence demonstrates the efficacy of this type of splint is only whilst the appliance is in use. This makes their prescription hard to justify given the risk of condylar remodeling and the development of an anterior open bite if used for long periods of time.

16.2 Physiotherapy

Active intervention with a physiotherapist has the potential to provide added benefit when used alongside self-exercise strategies. For all other sub-diagnoses of persistent TMD (myogenous and intra-articular), physiotherapy has the potential to reduce pain intensity and increase range of jaw opening. A strong association is found for physiotherapy providing short-term relief. Long-term benefit is not as consistently demonstrated; however, when prescribed appropriately, physiotherapy is unlikely to do harm, and so intermittent physiotherapy over the longer term may be appropriate. Physiotherapy provides the added benefit of promotion of engagement in self-management.

An appropriate physiotherapy regime will be assessed and prescribed by the physiotherapist on an individual basis. Active techniques include but are not confined to manual therapy, jaw exercises, cervical exercises, mandibular manipulation, postural training, cervical mobilisation and manipulation, and myofascial and cervical release. The main aims of active physiotherapy are to:

1. Increase the individual's awareness as to the cause of their symptoms
2. Achieve muscle relaxation
3. Reduce muscle hyper-activity and re-establish joint movement
4. Relieve muscle pain, spasm, and oedema
5. To enable return to normal function

Physiotherapy has the potential for benefit above any beyond "hands-on" care. Reassurance and patient education from an additional source to share consistent messages around the condition are a huge benefit. Physiotherapists can continually assess, moderate, and motivate individuals through a course of treatment promoting supported self-management practices maximising their potential benefit.

The process of referral for physiotherapy will vary between regions, and GDPs should liaise with local hospital or community physiotherapy centres to clarify. Some units may accept direct referral from GDPs, while in other areas, the GDP may need to correspond with the medical practitioners to request referral. Alternatively, patients may decide to access physiotherapy privately once potential benefits have been outlined to them.

16.3 Acupuncture

There is strong evidence that acupuncture reduces pain intensity for myogenous TMDs. When used as an adjunctive treatment with other TMD interventions (e.g. self-management, splint therapy), pain reduction is optimised. Acupuncture when done by correctly by trained individuals will do no harm. In the UK, not all regions offer acupuncture through the national health service, and enquiries should be made with local services as to the best route, should referral be required. As for acupuncture, patients may choose to directly access care through the private sector, and if so, an acupuncturist with specific experience with orofacial pain should be advised.

16.4 Pharmacological Management

In a small number of TMD cases, pharmacological management may be required. All such cases must involve interactive decision-making between the individual with TMD and their clinician. This discussion should take into consideration the risks, benefits, interactions, and potential adverse effects, specific to the individual, all of which should be discussed openly and documented fully.

16.5 Analgesics

Acute, short-lived TMD pain, either in isolation or as a “flare-up” of persistent TMD, can be significant, and so appropriate empathy and engagement with the individual are needed. In such instances, short-term use of over-the-counter NSAIDs, e.g. ibuprofen, may be advised, though evidence about this is equivocal. When advising NSAIDS, the additional use of paracetamol will reduce the total NSAID dose and therefore reduce the risk of negative NSAID side effects such as gastro-intestinal disturbance. Long-term analgesic use to manage TMD pain is not appropriate due to both adverse effects on the renal and gastrointestinal systems and also the risk of developing medication overuse headache if more than 15 days of simple analgesia use in 1 month.

Topical use of ibuprofen gel may benefit myogenous TMDs when applied to the affected musculature. Application of the gel in combination with massage to the affected muscle would optimise efficacy. Clinicians must advise extra-oral use, avoiding the eye area. Heat should not be applied directly after use, and the individual should complete a patch test on a small area of non-visible skin to rule out dermatological reaction 24 h prior to application.

16.6 Neuromodulatory Agents

Persistent pain conditions in other areas of the body can be managed with antidepressant (amitriptyline, duloxetine) and antiepileptic medications (gabapentin). The main neuromodulatory agents used for TMD and their most common side effects are shown in Table 2. Evidence for their benefit specifically with regard to TMD is more limited, but the concurrent off-licence use of such medications in appropriate cases, as part of a comprehensive specialist treatment plan, can provide additional benefit with regard to pain control and restoration of function. To be able to consent fully to treatment, patients must be made aware of the off-licence use for TMD and potential side effects of such medications. In 2019, gabapentin became a Class C, schedule 3 controlled drug in the UK, and this is consistent with other countries elsewhere in the world. Other countries will have equivalent guidelines to ensure that professionals prescribing gabapentin must make patients aware of the risk of

Table 2 Common side effects of neuromodulatory agents

Amitriptyline	Duloxetine	Gabapentin
Drowsiness	Anxiety	Anxiety
Confusion	Decreased appetite	Abnormal appetite
Restlessness	Dizziness	Confusion
Dry mouth	Drowsiness	Constipation
Arrythmias	Dry mouth	Cough
Fainting	GIT issues (Diarrhoea, constipation, nausea)	Dry mouth
Headache		Dependence

dependence and misuse and how to protect against this. Clinicians should be rigorous in their history taking, explore other options where appropriate, and prescribe appropriately.

16.7 Botulinum Toxin

Botulinum toxin (BTX) has been shown to modify pain processing, reduce muscle activity, inhibit the release of inflammatory mediators, and reduce central sensitisation. Despite these actions, clinical studies for the use of localised BTX for the management of muscular TMDs demonstrate equivocal results. Furthermore, contradictory and limited data on the potential for reduction in bone volume and hypertrophic bone proliferation when BTX was delivered to the muscles of mastication raise concern over its use long term. At present the clinical evidence base does not support routine use for TMD.

16.8 Surgical Intervention

Surgical intervention is restricted to intra-articular TMDs and degenerative joint disease only. Options include arthroscopy, arthrocentesis, arthroplasty, intra-articular infiltration of medicaments, or joint replacement and are discussed in more detail in Chapter "TMJ Surgery". All surgical interventions regardless of how well planned and conducted will result in a degree of morbidity, meaning surgical intervention is only appropriate as an end-stage therapy when all other treatments have been exhausted.

16.9 Changes to Management since Original Publication

In the decade since the original iteration of this book, TMD research has led to changing clinical practice. The clinical evidence base for a number of management strategies discussed in the original text has changed. Equivocal results for short-wave diathermy, ultrasound, and laser therapy have been shown over time, and although they may offer benefit to myofascial TMD, the certainty of the effect is low.

There is no clinical evidence base for the use of the tri-cyclic antidepressant dothiepin hydrochloride to manage persistent TMD in the literature, and its use has been superseded by amitriptyline or duloxetine, the preferred antidepressant medications for pain management in persistent myogenous TMD.

Historically, benzodiazepines such as diazepam and temazepam may have been prescribed for TMD due to their muscle relaxant properties. The evidence base for efficacy in TMD is poor, and given the potential for dependency, addiction, profound sedation, and respiratory depression, the risks do not outweigh the benefits in most occasions to justify usage.

Further Reading

Greene CS. The etiology of temporomandibular disorders: implications for treatment. J Orofac Pain. 2001;15:93–105; discussion 106.

Katzberg RW, Westesson PL, Tallents RH, Drake CM. Anatomic disorders of the temporomandibular joint disc in asymptomatic subjects. J Oral Maxillofac Surg. 1996;54(2):147–53.

Naeije M, te Veldhuis AH, te Veldhuis EC, Visscher CM, Lobbezoo F. Disc displacement within the human temporomandibular joint: a systematic review of a 'noisy annoyance'. J Oral Rehabil. 2013;40:139–58. https://doi.org/10.1111/joor.12016.

Schiffman EL, Ahmad M, Hollender L, et al. Longitudinal stability of common TMJ structural disorders. J Dent Res. 2017;96(3):270–6. https://doi.org/10.1177/0022034516679396.

Howick J, Moscrop A, Mebius A, et al. Effects of empathic and positive communication in healthcare consultations: a systematic review and meta-analysis. J R Soc Med. 2018;111(7):240–52. https://doi.org/10.1177/0141076818769477. http://www.linus-geisler.de/dp/dp04_listening.html.

Riley P, Glenny A-M, Worthington HV, Jacobsen E, Robertson C, Durham J, et al. Oral splints for temporomandibular disorder or bruxism: a systematic review. Br Dent J. 2020;228(3):191–7.

Zhang L, Xu L, Wu D, Yu C, Fan S, Cai B. Effectiveness of exercise therapy versus occlusal splint therapy for the treatment of painful temporomandibular disorders: a systematic review and meta-analysis. Ann Palliat Med. 2021;10(6):6122–32. https://doi.org/10.21037/apm-21-451. Epub 2021 May 10

Hamasaki H. Effects of diaphragmatic breathing on health: a narrative review. Medicine. 2020;7:65. https://doi.org/10.3390/medicines7100065.

Chang KL, Fillingim R, Hurley RW, Schmidt S. Chronic pain management: nonpharmacological therapies for chronic pain. FP Essentials. 2015;432:21–6.

Smith PS, Mosscrop D, Davies SJ, Sloan, Al-Ani Z. The efficacy of acupuncture in the treatment of temporomandibular joint myofascial pain: A randomised controlled trial. J Dent. 2007;35:259–67.

Michelotti A, et al. Home-exercise regimes for the management of non-specific temporomandibular disorders. J Oral Rehabil. 2005;32(11):779–85.

Wright EKG. Manual of temporomandibular disorders. 4th ed. Wiley- Blackwell; 2020.

Wänman A, Marklund S. Treatment outcome of supervised exercise, home exercise and bite splint therapy, respectively, in patients with symptomatic disc displacement with reduction: a randomised clinical trial. J Oral Rehabil. 2020;47(2):143–9.

Nicolakis P, et al. Effectiveness of exercise therapy in patients with myofascial pain dysfunction syndrome. J Oral Rehabil. 2002;29(4):362–8.

Magesty RA, et al. Oral health-related quality of life in patients with disc displacement with reduction after counselling treatment versus counselling associated with jaw exercises. J Oral Rehabil. 2021;48(4):369–74.

Beecroft E, Palmer J, Penlington C, Avery L, Aggarwal V, Chase M, Davies S, Gerber B, Jagger R, Harrison S, Horton M, Jones L, Kalantzis A, Lie S, McKenna G, McMillan R, Morton M, Murphy E, Renton T, Thayer T, Weden A, Durham J. Management of painful temporomandibular disorder in adults. NHS England Getting It Right First Time (GIRFT) and Royal College of Surgeons' Faculty of Dental Surgery; 2023. Available from: https://www.rcseng.ac.uk/dental-faculties/fds/publications-guidelines/clinical-guidelines/

TMJ Surgery

A. Kalantzis, Emma Beecroft, Stephen Davies, and Justin Durham

1 Introduction

A temporomandibular joint (TMJ) surgeon should be part of a multi-disciplinary team (MDT), rather than work in isolation as is sometimes the case in a general hospital. The MDT ideally will have specialist oral and maxillofacial surgeons, restorative dentists, dental therapists, physiotherapists, pain specialists and clinical psychologists. This will improve the chances of reaching the correct diagnosis and delivering the appropriate specialist therapy, therefore improving outcomes, patient experience and satisfaction. It will allow each specialist the time to concentrate on their field of expertise. For the surgeon, this is of utmost importance given the facts that the aetiology of temporomandibular disorders (TMD) are multifactorial and that the majority of patients can be managed by conservative measures. In addition, the members of an MDT are constantly learning from each other, so appropriate management pathways and clinical satisfaction are constantly improving.

The commonest reason for a referral to an oral surgery/oral and maxillofacial surgery unit in the UK, after dentoalveolar surgery, is TMD. Following first-line treatment in primary care as per guidelines, a substantial proportion of patients are

A. Kalantzis (✉)
Manchester University Hospitals Foundation Trust, Manchester, UK
e-mail: athanasios.kalantzis@mft.nhs.uk

E. Beecroft · J. Durham
School of Dental Sciences, Newcastle University, Newcastle upon Tyne, UK
e-mail: emma.beecroft@newcastle.ac.uk; Justin.Durham@newcastle.ac.uk

S. Davies
Division of Dentistry, University of Manchester, Manchester, UK
e-mail: stephen.j.davies@manchester.ac.uk

S. Davies et al. (eds.), *Temporomandibular Disorders in Primary Dental Care*,
BDJ Clinician's Guides, https://doi.org/10.1007/978-3-032-01301-9_6

referred to oral and maxillofacial surgery, with either myalgia or disc displacement with reduction (DDwR, clicking). Even if a patient suffers from both sub-types of TMD, potentially causing some diagnostic confusion, usually nothing more than explanation, reassurance and simple advice is needed. It is obvious that it is inappropriate and inefficient for a specialist TMJ surgeon to triage all these patients to discover the very few that would benefit from more invasive procedures. In summary, a wide team with complementary interests but a common treatment philosophy is needed for an effective regional service.

Classification of TMD has been discussed in earlier chapters. Broadly speaking, the patients presenting in a TMD clinic are likely to be suffering with one of four conditions: (i) myalgia, (ii) disc disorder, (iii) degenerative joint disease (previously known as osteoarthritis) or (iv) other/rarer pathologies. The Wilkes system [1], often used historically by surgeons to classify joints, should not be thought of as 'staging' in the sense of an inevitable progression from one stage to the next; this is at best an oversimplification. Wilkes I (disc displacement with reduction) requires no more than simple reassurance. Wilkes II is probably over-diagnosed, as in most cases, careful examination will reveal coexistence of Wilkes I with myalgia, both of which are very common as mentioned above. Truly symptomatic and painful disc displacement with reduction with or without intermittent locking is relatively rare and needs acute diagnostic skills (see earlier chapters and tips below). It may respond to simple non-invasive measures with the aim of reducing pain and preventing closed lock in young patients. Arthrocentesis may reduce pain in resistant cases.

Wilkes III (disc displacement without reduction with limited opening) often follows a period of clicking (Wilkes I) but is associated with a sudden reduction in mouth opening (around 25 mm for a typical patient in their early 20s), significant pain and ceasing of any joint noises. Although this may respond to early non-invasive measures, selected patients (e.g. younger adults with an acute lock) may have a quicker progress to less functional limitation with arthrocentesis. However, robust data suggest that remodelling of a displaced disc that has not reduced will occur in all age groups over 6–18 months returning to near-normal function with simple, supportive self-management techniques. Although patients are less likely to experience a closed lock the older they get (as the disc gets smaller), patients in their 30s or even 40s may still develop disc displacement without reduction, but as the point of obstruction typically moves further forward with age, their mouth opening will usually be >30 mm. Arthrocentesis is unlikely to improve the mouth opening (non-reducible disc) but may reduce arthrogenous pain.

Things get even more complicated once structural changes have occurred in the TMJ (Wilkes IV and V). One must remember that these are not necessarily the result of disc disorders, as osteoarthrosis and internal derangement may coexist even in a young patient. For some of these patients, some surgical intervention may become necessary if symptoms are not controlled with conservative measures and functions (diet and occlusion) are affected. For many years, the wide variety of conservative measures employed in the management of TMD was mirrored by a large number of open procedures for patients with predominantly articular symptoms and signs. However, long-term results from most of these procedures have been disappointing. In contrast, the favourable benefit vs risk profile of arthrocentesis (lysis and lavage) and total alloplastic joint replacement has contributed to these two procedures gradually gaining ground over all other TMJ interventions in the last three decades.

Box 1: TMJ/Condylar Disorders That Are Candidates for Surgical Intervention

- Disc displacement without reduction with limited opening (especially in younger adults)
- Degenerative joint disease (including following trauma and surgery)
- Ankylosis (e.g. following neonatal trauma or infection)
- Inflammatory arthropathies (rheumatoid arthritis, juvenile idiopathic arthritis, psoriatic arthritis)
- Condylar hyperplasia (transverse or vertical type)
- Condylar hypoplasia (hemifacial/craniofacial microsomia)
- Tumours (chondroma, osteoma, sarcoma, 2°)
- Idiopathic condylar resorption
- Synovial (osteo)chondromatosis
- Genetic disease

For some patients and health professionals, it is difficult to comprehend that in most cases, the scope of TMJ surgery will progress straight from a minimally invasive procedure such as arthrocentesis/arthroscopy to radical surgery (total joint replacement; TJR) without trying something 'simpler'. The perception is that there is nothing to lose and the patient may benefit from a less risky procedure. However, clinical experience (and, to a lesser extent, evidence) has shown that there is no 'simple' open TMJ procedure that gives predictable, good long-term outcomes in cases of objective pathology affecting the TMJ with high pain scores, limited mouth opening and poor function if myalgia TMD has been excluded as the primary pain. Furthermore, it is well documented that previous open surgery (especially multiple operations) leads to poorer outcomes if TJR is subsequently needed. Patients are likely to make different decisions once presented with this information.

It is apparent that the most critical part of the surgeon's role is identifying those patients that will benefit from surgery (Box 1). The use of current evidence and guidelines should supplement rather than become dogma over careful and meticulous clinical history and examination, leading to accurate and considered clinical judgement, which is discussed with the patient and shared decision-making engaged in. Without the correct diagnosis and appropriate patient counselling and consent, less-than-ideal outcomes and a poor patient experience and/or outcome are to be expected. Often, the most difficult challenge for the clinician is to differentiate between myogenous and arthrogenous pain and then identifying those cases of isolated arthrogenous pain which would benefit from surgical intervention. Other than direct palpation over the TMJ's and the masticatory muscles to see whether tenderness can be elicited, the compression test (a modification of Mahan's test), as described in Chapter "Examination and Diagnosis of Temporomandibular Disorders", may distinguish between two pains with different origins [2]. Essentially, the patient is asked to bite hard against two wooden spatulas with their back teeth on either side. Any ipsilateral pain elicited will be myogenous, whilst any contralateral pain will be arthrogenous. Any combination of results is possible depending on the patient's pathology. The test's specificity is high, which is very important in the context of its use. Its sensitivity however may be reduced by several factors, hence if doubt still exists, an injection of local anaesthetic block of the auriculotemporal nerve can be diagnostic (Fig. 1) [3].

The use of imaging in TMD patients is a matter of debate both from the perspective of justification for ionising imaging and also the high-false-positive and risk of confirmation bias with MRI if its ordering precludes careful examination [4]. It is important to understand that once a surgical intervention is considered, the

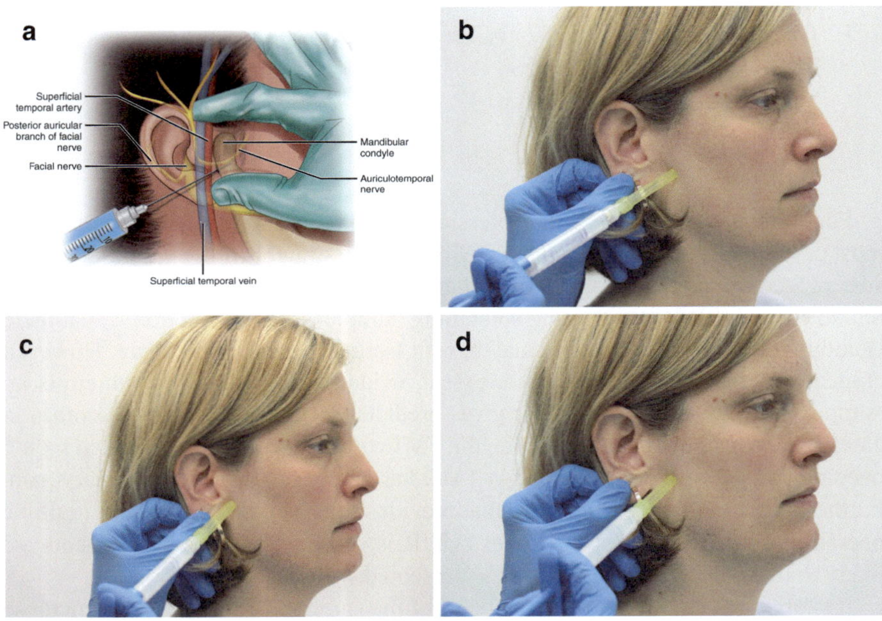

Fig. 1 Modified auriculotemporal block [3]. (**a**) Schematic of the anatomy of the area and needle position. Images B to D represent the needle positions to deliver the modified block. After cleaning the skin for an 'aseptic no-touch technique', a 35 mm 27G needle on an *aspirating* syringe is inserted (sheathed for model's safety in this image) just below the junction of ear lobe and tragus continuing anterosuperiorly until the posterior aspect of the condylar neck is encountered (**b**). Once the bone is contacted, reorientate the needle so it is advanced slightly more posteriorly and therefore medial to the condyle (**c**). Once it is past the condyle, reorientate again to a more anterior direction but now medial to the condyle, and advance a few more millimetres, (**d**) and *aspirate* prior to injection. The advantage of this approach is that it minimises the amount of facial nerve weakness caused by using this block for diagnostic (identifying arthrogenous from myogenous) or therapeutic (for arthrocentesis/arthroscopy) purposes

justification for obtaining an orthopantomogram may be much lower. In contrast, despite common misconception, an MRI scan may not be required for a routine case of disc displacement without reduction with limited opening, as the diagnosis is largely clinical in most cases. However, if proceeding to surgery, MRI might be advisable for confirmation. Some patients who need significant surgery involving hard tissues (including TJR) will need a CT or CBCT scan for accurate treatment planning. Nuclear bone scans are also useful in some cases.

2 Minimally Invasive Interventions

2.1 Arthrocentesis

Since described by Nitzan in 1991 [5], arthrocentesis has become the commonest intervention performed by TMJ surgeons for the treatment of arthrogenous TMD. Arthrocentesis is effective for reducing pain and improving mouth opening in acute disc displacement without reduction with limited opening in younger adults. In more established disc displacement without reduction with limited opening (in older adults) and/or degenerative joint disease, it is effective for pain reduction, which may only persist over the short term (months rather than years), and therefore, patients should be made aware it may not be a definitive solution and its outcomes can be unpredictable. Its benefits are achieved through pressure hydrolysis that breaks adhesions and through copious lavage that dilutes inflammatory mediators in the upper joint space.

Arthrocentesis can be performed under LA or GA. The classic technique involves the insertion of two needles. The two positions are termed anterior and posterior needle positions. The posterior position is placed first 10 mm anterior and 2 mm below a line starting at the middle of the tragus and travelling forward to the lateral canthus (Holmlund-Hellsing line [6]: see Fig. 2). The anterior position is placed by moving 20 mm along the same line from the tragus and then insertion 10 mm below it at that point.

When placing the posterior needle first, its insertion should aim slightly anteriorly and superiorly to a maximum insertion depth of up to 25 mm. This may be done with an active or passive opening of the joint if necessary. Accurate position of the needle tip in the upper joint space is confirmed by injecting up to 5 ml of saline (lysis), whereby a certain amount of resistance should be felt (as if trying to 'blow up a balloon'), the chin may protrude (unless significant adhesions exist) and most of the fluid returns back ('bounces back') to the syringe upon release of pressure if the joint capsule has enough elasticity. After insertion of the second needle in the anterior position (with outflow of saline confirming accurate position), irrigation (lavage) of 100–200 ml of saline through the joint is performed under pressure from the posterior needle position. The second needle is then removed, and any

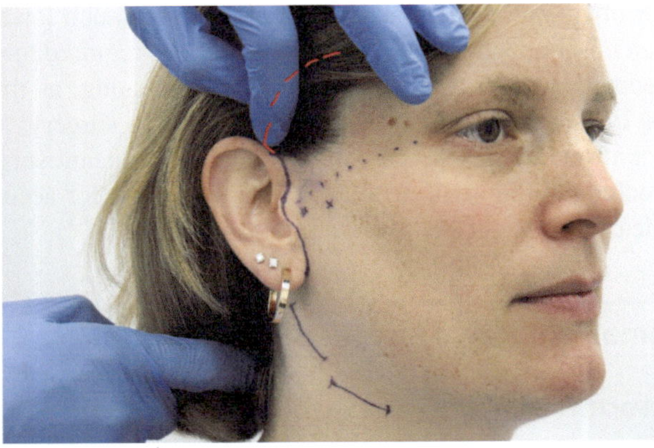

Fig. 2 Hellsing-Holmlund ('tragal-canthal line') line (dotted), arthrocentesis/arthroscopy points (two crosses inferior to dotted line), and common open surgical approaches marked up from superior to inferior: preauricular, retromandibular, submandibular all of which may be used in combination*. The Al-Kayat and Bramley extension of the preauricular would lie under the left hand of the operator in the picture and is indicted by the dotted red line. (*These are approximate indications of the positions/incisions and may vary dependent on anatomy of patient amongst other factors)

intra-articular medication is administered before the posterior needle is removed and any manipulation is performed.

Arthrocentesis is a simple and safe procedure; rarely complications may occur. These include:

- Facial nerve injury from repeated cannulation attempts (especially at the anterior site)
- Oedema from leakage of fluid out of the joint (especially if arthritic joints are repeatedly punctured)
- Damage to the ear from a posteriorly advanced needle
- Intracranial complications from perforation of the glenoid fossa (from forceful advancement of the needle through the 1-mm-thin bone separating the joint from the middle cranial fossa)
- Haematoma from injury of the external temporal artery
- Severe postoperative pain
- Needle breakage

Unsuccessful cannulation leads to repeated attempts that gradually increase the risk of complications and decrease the efficacy of the procedure. In the authors' experience, a maximum of three attempts should be undertaken for either needle before abandoning the procedure, or if a posterior needle is patent, consider a single-needle technique, using only this needle as described below.

Alternative techniques have been described in an attempt to make insertion of the anterior needle easier and safer especially in osteoarthritic and degenerative joints.

Most of these techniques involve moving the insertion point posteriorly and superiorly closer to the first needle, moving it away from the facial nerve. Some clinicians use a double-needle cannula to avoid a second puncture altogether. Furthermore, a single-needle technique where the joint is repeatedly filled with fluid and emptied actively or passively by opening and closing the mouth, respectively, has been shown to be as effective as the two-needle technique and can achieve effective and safe lysis of adhesions especially in arthritic joints where the two-needle technique may be more difficult.

Various irrigation fluids have been suggested for lysis and lavage. Some reports have suggested that Hartmann's solution (Ringer's lactate) may give better results than normal saline, as it is more physiological; however, given the purpose of the procedure and the small potential volume of the upper joint space (1.5–2 ml), it is difficult to argue the strength of the association. Furthermore, various amounts of fluid have been claimed as necessary for adequate dilution of inflammatory mediators, usually over 100 ml. Again, given the limited joint space, it is difficult to understand the necessity of volumes above 100 ml unless they are contributing to further lysis (under pressure), which could be achieved best before the second needle is inserted or by modifying the technique/pressure slightly. At the end of the procedure and before the last needle is removed, many clinicians administer a variety of medications intra-articularly. Corticosteroids (triamcinolone, depomedrone) may be effective in reducing inflammation, but should not be used repeatedly or routinely as they may promote condylar lysis. There is also some evidence supporting intra-articular hyaluronate and morphine injections, whilst platelet-rich plasma (PRP) may hold some promise for the future.

The evidence for the use of arthrocentesis versus non-invasive measures in the treatment of disc displacement without reduction with limited opening has been debated. A recent systematic review and meta-analysis [7] concluded that current evidence does not provide strong support for the use of arthrocentesis as first-line treatment for TMD. The only clear benefit of arthrocentesis was a small reduction in pain scores. However, significant heterogeneity between the studies, considerations about the accuracy of the specific diagnoses, concurrent treatments and other confounding factors complicating the study of invasive techniques in particular indicate that any evidence should be interpreted critically and must be used alongside clinical judgement. Therefore, although in the majority of cases non-invasive techniques will form the first-line treatment of closed lock and arthrogenous pain, close monitoring of response is imperative, and early referral for surgical opinion is important in selected cases. Some typical examples will be presented below.

Hypothetical example patient 1: A 20-year-old female presenting with acute pain over the right TMJ and limited mouth opening. She reports a 2-year history of a painless click from this joint that stopped 1 month previously. Since that time, she has had significant pain and limited mouth opening. On examination, she has a tender right TMJ, but no tenderness in the muscles of mastication. Compression test (modified Mahan's test) is positive for right arthrogenous pain. Mouth opening is 26 mm with lasting deviation to the right.

This is a typical case of disc displacement without reduction with limited opening (in a patient with pre-existing asymptomatic disc displacement with reduction). As the history of lock is short, the patient is young and they have no myogenic signs, early non-invasive measures (such as analgesia, stabilisation splint, manipulation, etc.) may work, but some may take significant time do so, whilst a small subset of patients may develop a chronic lock in the process. In contrast, patient 1 is likely to respond extremely well to early arthrocentesis, which can give a quick and very effective reduction in pain and return to a normal mouth opening. Therefore, for patients in this group, as illustrated by this case history, early referral to a specialist TMJ surgeon is appropriate.

Hypothetical example patient 2: A 25-year-old male presenting with pain in both preauricular areas and limited mouth opening. He has had persistent pain and intermittent self-resolving episodes of locking over the last 3 years but has not been able to open fully for the last 3 months. On examination, he has tender TMJs and muscles of mastication bilaterally. Compression test (modified Mahan's test) is positive for arthrogenous and myogenous pain bilaterally. Mouth opening is 28 mm without joint noises.

This is a case of disc displacement without reduction with limited opening + myalgia TMD. As the history, signs and diagnosis are more complex, there is certainly more justification in this scenario for starting with non-invasive measures. Arthrocentesis would not be expected to have a significant effect on the myogenous element of the condition unless this was purely secondary to the closed lock. Furthermore, patients with chronic myalgia have a higher risk of relapsing disc displacement without reduction with limited opening even if this is treated successfully with arthrocentesis. In conclusion, non-invasive measures (education, strong analgesia, heat, stabilisation splint, short course of diazepam [in acute presentation], amitriptyline, gabapentin or duloxetine) should be employed first, and if the patient does not fully respond, he should be referred for a surgical opinion, as at this age, the disc displacement should be reducible in the majority of cases. However, as stated, the risk of relapse even after successful treatment with arthrocentesis may be high, and the patient should receive advice regarding long-term self-management/physiotherapy with heat followed by mouth-opening exercises.

Hypothetical patient 3: A 38-year-old female presenting with worsening left-sided TMJ pain and stiffness. She has long-standing history of TMD, including a previous closed lock (disc displacement without reduction with limited opening) treated successfully with non-invasive measures almost 20 years previously. On examination, she has a tender left TMJ, but no tenderness in the muscles of mastication. Compression test (modified Mahan's test) is positive for left arthrogenous and myogenous pain. Mouth opening is 34 mm.

Despite the reasonable mouth opening, the diagnosis is again disc displacement without reduction with limited opening at least on the left side (see Introduction). Due to the chronicity of the condition, it is very likely that they may also have myalgia. It may be difficult to establish the condition of the contralateral joint if it currently has minimal symptoms and signs. Finally, the possibility of early degenerative joint disease in these cases should be explored. An early MRI of the TMJs in this case may be useful. Initially, non-invasive measures (education, analgesia, heat, stabilisation splint, amitriptyline gabapentin or duloxetine) should be employed, and if the patient does not fully respond, she should be referred for a surgical opinion. Arthrocentesis (or arthroscopy in this case) may be beneficial for reducing her pain score, but it is unlikely to improve her mouth opening.

The above examples highlight some of the difficulties of assessing the applicability and effectiveness of various measures in slightly different presentations of even a very specific diagnosis such as disc displacement without reduction with limited opening. The clinical decision may be influenced by patient age, severity of symptoms, concurrent diagnoses, chronicity, response to previous measures, access to services, clinician experience and patient preference. It is important that patients understand the potential benefits and risks of each therapy and make informed decisions. Arthrocentesis may improve mouth opening in selected patients and may be effective at reducing joint pain in a wide range of TMD with arthrogenous origin, thereby reducing the risk of escalating to open surgery. However, it offers little diagnostic value; when this is necessary along with the advantages of arthrocentesis, arthroscopy may be offered.

2.2 Arthroscopy

Arthroscopy is increasingly gaining popularity amongst TMJ surgeons despite the steep learning curve and initial expense of setting up the service. It involves the insertion of a scope through a small puncture in a similar location to the posterior insertion point for the first needle in the arthrocentesis technique. Visualisation of the upper joint space including the synovial lining and disc (position, fibrillations, perforation, adhesions) gives diagnostic advantages over arthrocentesis. A second puncture may be made anteriorly in a similar position to arthrocentesis' second needle anterior position in order to allow an outflow port for irrigation (lavage) or simple instrumentation (adhesiolysis). This forms the basis of Level I arthroscopy. The outcomes are similar to arthrocentesis for patients with anterior disc displacement without reduction, but arthroscopy has additional diagnostic benefits.

Level II and Level III arthroscopy involve the insertion of additional ports and the use of more complex equipment and techniques. This forms the basis of therapeutic arthroscopy with the advantage of avoiding open surgery in those patients resistant to more conservative measures. Level II arthroscopy involves the use of a second working port (instead of an irrigation needle at the second puncture site), thereby allowing for therapeutic interventions such as lysis, coblation, biopsy or lateral release. Level III arthroscopy typically involves three working/instrumentation ports that allow disc manipulation and joint surface reduction. Procedures may therefore include disc repositioning, discectomy and eminectomy. However, the expertise for such procedures is currently limited and used only in a small number of specialist centres.

Indications for arthroscopy might include:

- Disc displacement without reduction with limited opening (Wilkes III) in specific instances such as those noted in the recent Royal College of Surgeons of England guidelines (https://www.rcseng.ac.uk/-/media/FDS/Comprehensive-guideline-Management-of-painful-Temporomandibular-disorder-in-adults-March-2024.pdf)
- Degenerative joint disease (Wilkes IV)
- Inflammatory arthropathies
- Recurrent dislocation
- Uncertainty regarding diagnosis of TMJ pathology
- Need to confirm irreversible intra-articular pathology to justify escalation to TJR
- Need to sample tissue from the joint

Typically, a 1.9 mm arthroscope is used in the TMJ. For Level I and II arthroscopy, insertion points are as per arthrocentesis (see Fig. 2). The posterior port is inserted with the help of a trocar, which is then replaced with the scope for visualisation of the joint. The second sheath is introduced at the antero-lateral part of the upper joint space allowing irrigation or the introduction of an instrument. The joint is kept expanded and clear through constant irrigation. Important landmarks are identified, and the joint is examined for inflammation and loosening of the posterior disc attachment, perforation of the disc, adhesions, fibrillations and hyperaemia. Representative images are saved on the patient's records. Therapeutic procedures may be undertaken with the use of various instruments through the second port. More complex procedures, such as disc repositioning/plication, typically require additional small incisions or ports. Various techniques have been described, especially with regard to suturing/securing the disc posteriorly. Therapeutic arthroscopy is still highly specialised practice and detailed description of techniques is beyond the scope of this chapter. Irrespective of technique, the outcomes of arthroscopy in cases of painful anterior disc displacement without reduction (especially when treated early) seem to be at least equivalent to those of open surgery with the advantages of reduced complications and avoidance of the detrimental effects of repeated open surgery on the success of a future TJR (see below).

3 Open TMJ Surgery

3.1 Disc Surgery

As mentioned earlier in the chapter, it is now less common for this type of surgery to be conducted given advances in understanding in TMD but also the knowledge of the poor predictability of the outcomes of this type of open TMJ surgery. In addition, some of these procedures are gradually superseded by equivalent arthroscopic ones. If conducted, open disc surgery is usually performed in cases of anterior disc displacement without reduction.

Disc plication involves posterior repositioning of the disc after removal of some of the retrodiscal tissue.

Discopexy is a technique whereby the disc is freed up before being attached to the condyle with permanent sutures or a Mitek anchor pin.

Discectomy is usually performed when the disc is irreparable. The disc is removed, and the space is either left empty or replaced with ear cartilage, dermis-fat graft or temporalis fascia/muscle flap.

3.2 Bone Surgery

Arthroplasty (condyloplasty/condylar shave) is rarely performed, as outcomes are poor.

Condylectomy may be used in cases of condylar pathology. In cases of active condylar hyperplasia, early high condylectomy may be curative and prevent further deformity. In cases of ankylosis, reconstruction of the TMJ may be necessary, or a gap arthroplasty may suffice in children; ultimately, a total joint replacement is the most common outcome following condylectomy for most serious pathology including DJD.

Eminoplasty is usually performed to prevent TMJ subluxation or recurrent dislocation (open lock). Techniques include eminectomy (removal of the articular eminence), bone grafting (to augment the eminence) and Dautrey's procedure (down-fracturing of the zygomatic arch).

4 Total Alloplastic TMJ Replacement

End stage TMJ disease may be due to varying arthritides, but many other conditions may lead to destruction of the normal TMJ structures including the condyle (see Box 1). The clinical appearance of end-stage degenerative TMJ disease (Wilkes V) does not correspond with patient age, nor does it necessarily closely relate to radiological findings as already discussed. Although many publications have provided absolute or relative indications for reconstruction of the TMJ, especially with a total joint replacement (TJR), each individual case should be considered based on the specific diagnosis, prognosis, disease-specific quality of life and likelihood of improving the patient's quality of life in the long term with an acceptable risk profile.

As mentioned earlier, the first step is to establish that the patient's symptoms are originating from the joint. This should be done even when advanced degenerative joint disease or other arthritic processes have been demonstrated on a scan for reasons already described. The relationship between myogenous and arthrogenous pain may be complex. Often in chronic cases, there will be an element of both, and the clinician must try to elicit which is the predominant feature (the primary 'familiar pain' and complaint of the patient). Occasionally, repeated examinations may be necessary, as is careful review of the history. One must also consider that chronic joint pain may lead to associated limitation of opening through myogenous pain. It is therefore unsurprising that concentrating on treatment modalities that target one part of this finely balanced system only is not likely to give satisfactory results.

Once the pain has been confirmed as primarily arthrogenous (see introduction of this chapter) and the diagnosis has been specified, the patient symptoms and clinical findings should be recorded in detail. Only then can a decision be made on the likelihood of surgery improving the patient's condition. This will depend on the severity of the symptoms and signs.

The likely findings (and outcomes) in a typical candidate for TJR are as follows:

1. *Pain*: typically, a pain score of 6–8/10 (expected to be reduced to 1–3/10 after TJR).
2. *Limited mouth opening:* typically <30 mm due to joint pain/inflammation, adhesions or other pathology (expected to be ~35 mm on average after TJR, but without protrusion or contralateral excursion).
3. *Poor dietary score*: typically ~5/10 (expected to improve to 9-10/10 with TJR).
4. *Deranged occlusion* (anterior open bite, retrognathia, asymmetry): simultaneous correction of orthognathic and TMJ/condylar anomaly.

Box 2: Indications for TJR*

- TMJ or condylar pathology
  - Inflammatory, degenerative or 2° arthritis
  - Absence/loss of TMJ structures or ankylosis
- Symptoms of:
  - Pain
  - Limited opening
  - Difficulty eating
  - +/– altered occlusion (AOB, retrognathia, asymmetry)
- Failure of other treatments (conservative or surgical, including previous TJR)

*At least one indication in all three major categories should be satisfied.

Box 3: Risks/Complications of TJR

- Bleeding (transfusion, external carotid artery ligation): 3%
- Infection (usually leading to removal of implant): 2–3%
- Facial nerve weakness: <2% (up to 30% temporary)
- Numbness (auriculotemporal nerve): 14%
- Malocclusion/Malposition: 1%
- Pain/Swelling/Irritation: 1%
- Dislocation 1%
- Heterotopic bone/scar formation 1%
- Hypersensitivity, fractures, loosening, hearing loss: <1%

The indications for TJR are summarised in Box 2, whilst the risks are listed in Box 3.

Patient selection is key. It is imperative that those factors that may have an adverse effect on outcomes are recognised so that the patients who are less likely to do well with TJR are familiar with the risks:

- Medically and immunologically compromised patients are not likely to cope well with a prolonged operation, and the risk of implant infection may be high.
- Multiple previous open operations increase the difficulty of the procedure, decrease the efficacy of TJR and significantly increase complication rates.
- Surgeon experience is almost certainly a factor partly through its influence on operating time.
- Patients with less joint damage/degeneration have higher incidence of chronic postoperative pain after TJR [8].
- Other risk factors include:
  - Chronicity
  - Young age
  - Female sex
  - High BMI
  - Opioid analgesia
  - Psychosocial problems

Although there are no absolute contraindications, because of the extent of the surgery and the risks involved, appropriate consent and occasionally tertiary opinion should be sought.

The literature supporting the two main systems currently in use covers well over 2000 cases, many of which exceed 20 years of follow-up. It is now beyond doubt that TJR is a very effective procedure in carefully selected patients. Mercuri [9] and Gupta [10] have independently demonstrated a significant improvement in overall quality of life after TJR. Patient satisfaction has been shown at >95%. The National

Institute for Health and Care Excellence (NICE) in the UK has recommended that current evidence on efficacy and safety supports the use of TJR provided that:

- Arrangements are in place for clinical governance and audit
- Decisions are made in a multi-disciplinary specialist team environment
- All alternative therapies have been considered
- Finally, specialist training should be in place [11]

Prior to the introduction of alloplastic TMJ replacement, the main option for reconstruction of the condyle and TMJ was autologous bone grafts. Costochondral (rib) graft remains a viable option for growing children (see below) as are free vascularised flaps in adults on certain occasions. However, the relative technical ease, safety, predictability and long-term success of alloplastic implants have transformed the reconstructive surgery of the TMJ, especially in the last quarter of a century once the lessons from knee and hip joint surgery were applied.

The Vitek-Kent (Proplast-Teflon) prosthesis was the first to be widely used throughout the 1980's, but despite encouraging early results, outcomes turned out to be very disappointing and devastating in some patients primarily due to severe foreign body giant cell reactions. Another popular prosthesis in the 1990s was the Christensen metal-on-metal device, which had poor wear properties (fatigue) and subsequent particularisation (metalosis). Some of the early prostheses were available for hemiarthroplasty. However, it is now considered that total joint reconstruction of the fossa and condyle gives better and more stable long-term outcomes.

The ideal materials for joint reconstruction will be biocompatible and stable, withstand load and allow for an aseptic surgical technique. A wrought material such as titanium has most of these properties, hence, presents itself as the ideal material for the ramus/condylar part of the joint. Cobalt/chrome/nickel alloy is normally used on the articular surface of the condyle due to superior wear properties. Patients with known allergy to cheap jewellery should have a 'pure' titanium condylar prosthesis, and there is a consideration for the need for patch testing prior to use of an alloy-based TJR. There is still insufficient evidence as to whether the lifespan of a pure titanium implant would be significantly reduced. Ultra-high-molecular-weight (UHMW) polyethylene has emerged as the ideal material for the upper (fossa) part of the prosthesis due to its high tensile strength with little fragmentation. These materials had been used in orthopaedic surgery for decades.

For over two decades now, the two dominant prostheses for TJR have been the custom-fitted TMJ Concepts system (popularised by Mercuri [9]) and the Zimmer Biomet custom-fitted or stock device (popularised by Quinn [12]). These systems, using the current and accepted standard materials, have been extremely successful and safe in long-term studies, as already discussed. Recent comparative studies have shown no differences in outcomes between the two main companies or between custom and stock prostheses [13, 14]. However, where finances and time constraints allow, custom-fitted prostheses have gained wide popularity amongst surgeons even for routine cases. At the time of writing, there are more than 30 TJR systems in use or in development, as the popularity of the procedure is predicted to grow in the next decade or two at least [15].

The process for obtaining custom TJR(s) starts with a detailed discussion of the patient-specific expected outcomes versus risks of the procedure and ruling out all alternatives in an MDT setting. Once the patient has given informed consent, funding has been confirmed and allergy tests have been considered (e.g. targeted testing suggested by Mercuri [16]), then a fine-cut CT of the facial skeleton (TJR protocol) is obtained with the patient advised to keep the teeth gently in the planned occlusion. If this is not possible and the occlusion is going to change following the procedure, then models of the teeth fixed in the desired occlusion, along with records of the current occlusion, should be sent with the scans. Alternatively, 3D scans of the models or intraoral scans may be sent. The scan data needs to be accompanied by a prescription form of what is required and any other relevant information (e.g. metal allergies). Preliminary designs need to be approved by the surgeon before the implants go into production. In cases where the TMJ/condylar pathology has caused significant deformity and abnormal occlusion, combined TJR and orthognathic surgery is often required. The 3D planning and design is then more elaborate, as is the hardware used, including cutting guides and occasionally custom plates for all osteotomies, with increasing costs, which might take these options beyond the scope of some services around the world.

Surgery usually involves dual access from above (preauricular TMJ approach with Al-Kayat and Bramley [17] modification [temporal extension]) and from below (modified retromandibular approach) to avoid all the branches of the facial nerve (Fig. 2).

Once the condyle is removed and enough space is created in the fossa, using cutting guides in both cases, if necessary, the fossa element of the joint is fitted and fixed with four or five screws followed by fitting of the condylar element with a couple of screws until good positioning and occlusion are confirmed before the remaining bicortical screws are placed in the ramus. Good aseptic technique and avoidance of mouth-skin contamination is paramount to avoid implant infection and failure. If bilateral coronoidectomies have been performed along with TJRs (e.g. in cases of coronoid hyperplasia or extremely restricted mouth opening), the risk of immediate postoperative dislocation is considerable; hence, some precautions need to be taken for a few days (elastic IMF with braces or use of bandages). Patients are monitored closely on regular intervals as per guidelines and clinical governance requirements (discussed above).

5 Paediatric TMJ Surgery

TMD may affect teenagers or rarely children, but symptoms are usually mild and self-limiting. Parents of small children may complain of loud tooth grinding during the night, but this is common and usually of no consequence. Myalgia TMD may be seen in childhood and adolescence, but symptoms are usually well controlled with simple measures. Disc displacement with reduction may also be identified in adolescence, and simple reassurance should suffice along with some advice on unlocking manoeuvres (see Chapter "Management") if symptoms were to progress with episodes of pain and intermittent locking.

However, one should be mindful of young patients with persistent symptoms that do not conform to the typical patterns of TMD, especially when they exhibit primarily arthrogenous signs and some facial deformity, asymmetry or malocclusion. In these patients, the cause may be a congenital, inflammatory or other pathology affecting the TMJ and condyle, leading to abnormal development and subsequent deformity and dysfunction. Some of these conditions, for which surgical opinion should be sought, are listed in Box 4.

Box 4: Causes of TMJ/Condylar Pathology and/or Deformity in Children

- Congenital; condylar (+/− TMJ and facial) hypoplasia
  - Hemifacial/craniofacial microsomia (HFM)
  - Mandibulofacial dysostosis, e.g. Treacher Collins syndrome (TCS)
  - Pierre Robin syndrome (PRS)
- Developmental; condylar hyperplasia
  - Horizontal and vertical growth vectors (and associated deformities)
- Traumatic (condylar fracture ➔ ankylosis)
- Infective (infective arthritis ➔ ankylosis)
- Inflammatory (e.g. juvenile rheumatoid/idiopathic arthritis [JIA])
- Idiopathic (idiopathic condylar resorption [ICR])
- Genetic/metabolic (e.g. mucopolysaccharidosis, fibrous dysplasia)

At least 50% of patients with *JIA* will exhibit symptoms or signs of TMJ involvement, and opinion from a TMD specialist may be requested by the paediatric rheumatologist. Occasionally, the TMJ may be the first joint affected, and acute diagnostic skills may be needed. The patient will often have well-localised arthrogenous pain and restricted mouth opening, not conforming to history, age-profile or clinical findings typical of disc displacement without reduction with limited opening. An MRI with contrast will establish the severity of TMJ involvement, depending on level of joint effusion, synovial enhancement and condylar erosion. The first line of approach is to step up the patient's systemic therapy, often adding (or increasing the dose of) a biologic-type disease-modifying anti-rheumatoid drug (DMARD) such as infliximab. If the TMJ symptom control remains poor, the rheumatologist will often ask the TMD specialist for additional treatment such as an intra-articular steroid injection. This may be effective; however, the long-term benefits are questionable, whilst as already mentioned, there is emerging evidence that repeated steroid injections may cause condylar lysis or heterotopic bone formation. The authors would recommend considering a maximum of two doses of intra-articular steroids only in patients with well-established and poorly controlled rheumatoid disease affecting the TMJ and causing significant disability due to pain and restricted mouth opening. There is some evidence that intra-articular tumour-necrosis factor (TNF) inhibitors (such as infliximab) may be more effective than steroids. When assessing adolescents with JIA, other types of TMD (e.g. myalgia TMD or disc displacement without reduction with limited opening), possibly predisposed by the original dysfunction from the arthritis, should be considered. These conditions must be diagnosed and treated on their own merits, i.e. with physiotherapy, exercises, splint therapy or arthrocentesis.

Open surgery should have a limited role in JIA. This is because JIA affecting the condyle has a good prognosis if detected early and managed with methotrexate along with biologics. Young children who have not responded well to therapy or have been diagnosed late may suffer with significant clockwise deformity of the mandible and compromised airway. Every effort to control the disease and stabilise the joint should be made before advancing the mandible with conventional orthognathic techniques or distraction osteogenesis (depending on age and/or severity). In older children, especially those with persisting TMJ symptoms, TJRs may be a better option (see below).

Idiopathic condylar resorption (ICR) is a rare condition, which may present spontaneously in adolescents or after orthodontic treatment. The association with orthodontic treatment may be due to confounding factors. More importantly, ICR may occur after orthognathic surgery, especially following a large advancement of the mandible in a patient with the following risk factors:

- Female
- Teenager
- Class II
- High mandibular plane angle
- Pre-existing TMD (internal derangement)
- Low BMI

The aetiopathogenesis is likely to be complex and according to Wolford includes the following:

- Hormones mediate biochemical changes within the TMJ
- Hyperplasia of the synovial tissues
- Production of destructive substrates that initiate breakdown of the ligaments that normally support and stabilise the articular disc
- Disc becomes anteriorly displaced
- Synovial tissue then assumes a position around the head of the condyle
- Resorption occurring in the subcondylar bone without destruction of the fibrocartilage on the condylar head and roof of the fossa (unlike an inflammatory disease)
- Progress until the entire condylar head has been resorbed.

- Remission
- Excessive joint loading (i.e. parafunctional habits, trauma or orthognathic surgery) can reinitiate the resorption process later in life

Clinically, the patient presents with progressive worsening of occlusion and facial appearance (anterior open bite, retrognathia and retrogenia), often with little or no pain. Orthopantomogram and serial lateral cephalograms are useful, but the gold standard is a contrast MRI; this should demonstrate a small/short condyle with normal fibrocartilage, increased joint space full of synovial tissue and anterior disc displacement. Wolford and Cardenas have suggested a treatment protocol for ICR depending on the level of condylar destruction [18]. Essentially, if there is adequate condyle, they recommend open TMJ surgery for synovectomy, disc repositioning with Mitek anchor (or disc graft if the disc is not salvageable) and orthognathic surgery (including anticlockwise rotation, which they claim to be stable in conjunction with the recommended TMJ surgery). If the condyle however is unsalvageable, the patient needs reconstructive surgery with either a bone graft or TJR (see below).

There is a lot of conflicting and weak evidence relating to the *association of TMD and orthognathic surgery* [19]. Orthognathic deformities are not a significant factor for TMDs. Some exceptions may include Class II patients with deep bite (perhaps due to habitual anterior posturing of the mandible leading to early disc displacement and occasionally painful parafunction of the lateral pterygoid muscles) and condylar hyperplasia (also associated with disc displacement and occasionally myofascial pain). Equally, orthognathic treatment is not strongly linked to changes in TMDs. However, patients are more likely to improve, especially those with Class II deep bite deformities as above [20]. Class III patients who remain in heavy Class III elastics and limited opening for a prolonged period after surgery may experience worsening symptoms of TMD at least in the short term, probably due to reduced function of the joints. Orthognathic treatment is not contraindicated in TMD, but acute or severe problems must be addressed before elective therapies where possible, as already discussed.

Congenital disorders affecting the condyle and TMJ (such as various syndromes mentioned in Box 4) or acquired disorders (such as TMJ ankylosis) lead to underdevelopment of the mandible and TMJ structures. These may be unilateral or bilateral and can be graded using the Pruzansky classification (1969) [21], which was modified by Kaban in its currently used form (1988) [22]:

- 1: Small mandible
- 2A: Very small, abnormal ramus/condyle—functioning TMJ
- 2B: As above, but no functioning TMJ
- 3: Absent ramus/condyle/TMJ

This classification was initially devised for patients with HFM (the commonest head and neck syndrome after cleft lip and palate and probably widely underdiagnosed); however, it may be applied to any case of mandibular hypoplasia. The importance of this classification system is that it guides treatment decisions as below:

- 1 (e.g. mild to moderate cases of PRS)—non-surgical management or orthognathic surgery after completion of growth
- 2A (e.g. severe PRS [very small mandible], HFM, mild mandibulofacial dysostosis cases [such as TCS], ankylosis [leading to airway obstruction from retrognathia])—distraction osteogenesis (DO) of the mandibular body to improve airway
- 2B (moderate mandibulofacial dysostosis cases)—usually DO not an option; condylar reconstruction is necessary (see discussion below regarding bone grafting versus alloplastic reconstruction)
- 3 (severe mandibulofacial dysostosis cases)—more extensive reconstruction needed of ramus/condyle and fossa; the patient is likely to be dependent on tracheostomy for airway control

Whatever the cause of TMJ or condylar pathology in early life, retrognathia and limited mouth opening often soon ensue. In severe cases, these may result in airway compromise. Lower facial asymmetry and malocclusion may also be prominent features leading to dietary difficulties and cosmetic concerns. The main priorities for a maxillofacial surgeon in order of importance are:

1. *Airway.* Establish obstructive sleep apnoea (OSA) with formal sleep study (rather than simple overnight pulse oximetry); treat with anterior movement of the mandible/chin to open airway (DO of posterior mandibular body is a very useful technique but needs a 'posterior stop' [stable joint] to achieve aim; otherwise, condylar/TMJ reconstruction is needed [see below]); aim is to avoid tracheostomy (or decannulate), which improves health and QoL.
2. *Mouth opening.* Remove ankylosis, coronoid process hyperplasia (CPH) and other treatable causes of MMO restriction (see below); this has an impact on the airway, in particular access during general anaesthesia.
3. *Facial symmetry and aesthetics.* This is understandably often an unspoken but significant concern for parents, especially for children of school age, due to fear of psychosocial consequences; surgery (e.g. DO) can be very beneficial.
4. *Occlusion and diet.* Aim for as close relationship as possible between upper and lower arches; disappointingly, this does not usually improve oral intake in infants with congenital disorders in the short term, and in some cases, a significant 'improvement' of a severe malocclusion in older children may actually decompensate a previously well-adapted masticatory and swallowing function; therefore, expectations in this respect must be tempered.

As mentioned previously, the syndromic mandible may exhibit severe deficiency or absence of the condyle, ramus and TMJ (Pruzansky/Kaban 2b or 3). In these cases, reconstruction of the posterior mandible and occasionally the glenoid fossa is necessary, to improve the airway and re-establish function. Autogenous reconstruction with costochondral graft has been the gold standard in the growing patient for some time. Typically, the contralateral sixth rib is harvested (or fifth and seventh ribs if bilateral reconstruction is necessary), keeping 1 cm of cartilage and the periosteum/perichondrium around the junction to prevent separation. Access to the facial skeleton is as per TJR, and the graft is fixed to the posterior mandible, positioning the cartilage in the fossa. Intermaxillary fixation of 5–6 weeks should be followed by gradual mobilisation to avoid ankylosis. Fat grafting in the TMJ and the use of a wafer that increases occlusal height by 2–3 mm during IMF may be used for the same purpose. However, outcomes may be unpredictable, especially in terms of growth, and revision surgery is common [23, 24]. Vascularised free flaps (e.g. fibula or iliac crest) may be used in cases where a significant amount of tissue is missing or lost, or radiotherapy may be needed (e.g. oncological reconstruction). DO has been suggested for reconstruction of the TMJ, but complications may be expected, including technical issues with vector. Alloplastic reconstruction with an early or even temporising (for younger children) TJR is emerging as a safer and more predictable solution than autogenous bone, where access and financial constraints are not limiting factors.

Mandibular fractures are the most common facial injuries in children, and the condyle is the commonest site of fracture within the mandible. Unlike in adults, the commonest type of condylar fracture is diacapitular, i.e. it is the condylar head rather than the neck that breaks. This may not be evident on plain radiographs or orthopantomogram. Furthermore, even if there is no fracture of the jaw, there may still be articular damage with joint effusion or haemarthrosis. The articular disc may be damaged or displaced. The patient will experience pain, difficulty opening the mouth and occasionally malocclusion (especially if there are other fractures of the mandible). Paediatric condylar fractures are almost always treated without surgery. A short period of IMF may be useful for condylar neck fractures (seen in older children) that cause mild malocclusion. All other patients should get strong analgesia and encouraged to mobilise early in order to maintain good function, which should promote continuing growth and symmetry, and prevent ankylosis of the TMJ.

Ankylosis may result from any injury to the TMJ (especially in neonates and toddlers) including trauma, surgery or infective arthritis (e.g. secondary to acute mastoiditis). It needs to be differentiated from trismus or other causes of severe limitation of MMO. The history and a CT scan are usually diagnostic. Patients will have limited (if fibrous tissue still separates the condyle and fossa) or no mobility of the mandible, and growth on the affected side (and to some extend overall) will arrest. Severe retrognathia and inability to open the mouth amongst other problems may cause significant OSA and anaesthetic (airway access) concerns. Treatment involves removing the ankylotic bone from the TMJ and reconstructing the joint. Traditionally, this was done with a rib graft, but increasingly, TJR is seen as a more predictable option even for the paediatric patient. TJR is now considered the definitive treatment of choice for boys from 15 years and girls from 13–14 years [25]. It may also be the best temporising measure for children 8–12 years old, who will most likely need the implant replaced as part of an orthognathic plan after completion of growth. For younger children (who typically develop sleep apnoea early even with unilateral ankylosis), the author's preferred technique is to perform DO of the posterior mandibular body in order to bring the chin forward, improving the airway, cosmesis and subsequent function and increasing the bone stock. Release of ankylosis and temporalis interposition flap is performed 2 months later, at the time of the distractor removal. Long-term physiotherapy is an integral part of the success of any technique in early life. The aim is to maintain function, minimise surgery and scarring and optimise growth, with a view to progressing to TJR either at completion of growth or earlier if necessary (e.g. recurrence of OSA, severe asymmetry or cosmetic concerns). Extensive new evidence supports this focus on 'function rather than reconstruction' approach in paediatric ankylosis, and the use of DO before ankylosis release, for improved outcomes and reduced risk of re-ankylosis.

Just as with adults, extra-articular causes of mouth opening restriction (other than pain of myogenous origin) should always be considered, when the cause is not obvious and, in particular, when the limitation is severe. Infection (e.g. acute abscess involving the masticator space) is not uncommon in adolescence, and the origin is usually dental. A tumour invading the masticatory muscles will have the same effect, albeit less acute and usually not associated with other symptoms of infection including severe pain. Mouth cancer is rare in children, but sarcomas of soft or hard tissues around the jaw may present with trismus. Children who have had radiotherapy for such tumours are likely to suffer with severe trismus, which is difficult to treat. Scarring from previous surgery on and around the jaw may have similar effects. Myositis ossificans is a rare condition that may affect the masticatory muscles, causing trismus, which only gets worse with further surgery.

One of the commonest causes of extra-articular restriction of mouth opening is *coronoid process hyperplasia (CPH)*. This may develop in any patient who has been subject to prolonged restriction of full TMJ function (of any aetiology) during early childhood. CPH is characterised by the impingement of the elongated coronoid process on the posterior surface of the zygomatic body with mouth opening. The coronoid process of the mandible is normally shorter than the condylar process and usually less than 15 mm in height from the base of the sigmoid notch. However, in cases of CPH, the coronoid is longer than the condyle. With 3D CT, it is easy to visualise the CPH and the relationship with the zygoma. In a meta-analysis, McLoughlin et al. [26] found that the condition most often affected adolescent men and was more commonly bilateral. In a systematic review, Mulder et al. [27] reported that the main clinical symptom in all cases was a slow, progressive reduction in MMO. The mean MMO at presentation was 16 mm.

In terms of the aetiopathogenesis, CPH may be a feature of any condition adversely affecting TMJ function in early life, as mentioned above. Progressive mandibular hypomobility therefore appears to be not only the result of CPH but also the original causative factor. TMJ pathology leading to CPH includes trauma, infection, arthritis, radiotherapy, chronic non-infective (juvenile) osteomyelitis (CNO) and other causes of fibrous or bony ankylosis during growth. However, a true causative effect or mechanism has not been clearly established. Some theories emphasise the interplay of hypo-activity, myostatic contracture, inflammatory response and fibrosis of the temporalis muscle and the interaction of the temporalis with the suprahyoid muscles. However, there is limited evidence behind any of these theories. Some form of pathologic distraction osteogenesis of the coronoid process seems to be taking place as part of the pathogenesis. The shortening of the condyle and mandibular ramus in cases of condylar pathology leading to an upward migration of a coronoid process, the growth of which may not be at all reliant on the condylar growth centre, must also be considered as a contributory factor. Moreover, in the majority of cases, there also appears to be true hyperplasia of the coronoid. In mucopolysaccharidosis, the coronoids can reach enormous proportions both in height and width, and it is speculated that other factors such as the dysostosis multiplex seen in these patients or soft tissue factors may also play a role.

The treatment of CPH is surgery as the restriction is principally caused by mechanical obstruction. Two types of surgery may be performed: coronoidotomy or coronoidectomy. During a coronoidotomy, the coronoid is sectioned at the base usually via an intra-oral approach at the retro-molar region and left in situ. In this situation, it usually migrates superiorly due to temporalis muscle contraction. A coronoidectomy involves stripping of the temporalis muscle from the coronoid and subsequent removal of the coronoid via an intra-oral approach. Extremely large processes may need an extra-oral (temporal) approach in order to deliver the osteotomised bone. This is often the case in patients with mucopolysaccharidosis, due to the size of the coronoids. Either procedure has its respective advantages and disadvantages, with coronoidotomy being easier to perform, but possibly carrying a higher risk of recurrence. Coronoidectomy is the preferred method for most OMF surgeons. Coronoidectomy may also be performed in cases of restricted MMO where CPH is not a feature, for example, patients with muscle hyperactivity of any cause. However, the results are not usually as satisfactory as in CPH. Post-operative physiotherapy is considered to play an important role in maintaining and increasing the MMO. Active and passive stretching exercises with or without the use of spatulas, trismus screw or TheraBite© should be used.

One final condition that is worth discussing here is *chronic non-infective osteomyelitis (CNO)* of the jaw. This is a recurring, sclerosing form of osteomyelitis usually affecting one ramus of the mandible in children and adolescents, leading to painful enlargement of the bone as well as the surrounding soft tissues during exacerbations. Oedema and chronic inflammation of the masticatory muscles may progress to masseter and pterygoid hypertrophy in some patients with resultant trismus. Clinical presentation typically raises suspicion of infective osteomyelitis or bone malignancy, leading to repeated (but unnecessary) operations for histology and microbiology samples, which are non-specific. CT scan shows lytic and sclerotic areas, expansion and often periosteal reactive bone apposition (Gare's osteomyelitis). ESR is usually elevated. CNO is thought to be an auto-inflammatory condition and part of the chronic recurrent multifocal osteomyelitis (CRMO) spectrum [28]. However, despite some reports in the literature, most cases of mandibular CNO appear to be unifocal. First-line treatment consists of strong long-term NSAIDs such as indomethacin. This usually prevents recurrent painful soft tissue swellings, but bone swelling does not reduce. Early liaison with paediatric rheumatology is necessary for consideration of full-body MRI scan (to rule out CRMO) and second-line medical therapy consisting usually of bisphosphonates (such as IV pamidronate), which are both effective and safe in children, and may offer advantages in bone remodelling and hence cosmetic outcomes [29]. Escalation should be considered in patients with:

- Severe symptoms or deformity
- Poor response to indomethacin
- Intolerance to NSAIDs
- Persistent disease past the age of 18
- Multifocal disease

As already described, direct involvement of the masticatory muscles and occasionally the condyle may cause symptoms that mimic TMD. In adolescents, TMD may coexist with CNO, the latter being a contributing or precipitating factor. In such cases, it is important that pain from TMD is differentiated from CNO relapse and does not lead to unnecessary escalation of treatment as above. It is therefore important that patients are managed in a multi-disciplinary team led by a paediatric OMF Surgeon, who has a good understanding of paediatric TMDs and established links with paediatric rheumatology.

References

1. Wilkes CH. Internal derangements of the temporomandibular joint. Pathological variations. Arch Otolaryngol Head Neck Surg. 1989;115(4):469–77.
2. Mahan, P.E. and C.C. Alling, Facial pain. 3rd . Vol. 23. 1991, Philadelphia: Lea & Febiger.
3. Donlon WC, Truta MP, Eversole LR. A modified auriculotemporal nerve block for regional anesthesia of the temporomandibular joint. J Oral Maxillofac Surg. 1984;42(8):544–5.
4. Petersson A. What you can and cannot see in TMJ imaging--an overview related to the RDC/TMD diagnostic system. J Oral Rehabil. 2010;37(10):771–8.
5. Nitzan DW, Dolwick MF, Martinez GA. Temporomandibular joint arthrocentesis: a simplified treatment for severe, limited mouth opening. J Oral Maxillofac Surg. 1991;49(11):1163–7. discussion 1168-70
6. Holmlund A, Hellsing G. Arthroscopy of the temporomandibular joint. An autopsy study. Int J Oral Surg. 1985;14(2):169–75.
7. Hu Y, Liu S, Fang F. Arthrocentesis vs conservative therapy for the management of TMJ disorders: a systematic review and meta-analysis. J Stomatol Oral Maxillofac Surg. 2023;124(1s):101283.
8. Valdes AM, et al. Inverse relationship between preoperative radiographic severity and postoperative pain in patients with osteoarthritis who have undergone total joint arthroplasty. Semin Arthritis Rheum. 2012;41(4):568–75.
9. Mercuri LG, Edibam NR, Giobbie-Hurder A. Fourteen-year follow-up of a patient-fitted total temporomandibular joint reconstruction system. J Oral Maxillofac Surg. 2007;65(6):1140–8.
10. Gupta B, Ahmed N, Sidebottom AJ. Quality of life outcomes one year after replacement of the temporomandibular joint using a modified SF36 questionnaire. Br J Oral Maxillofac Surg. 2020;58(3):304–8.
11. NICE. Total prosthetic replacement of the temporomandibular joint. Interventional procedures guidance [IPG500]. 2014. Available from: https://www.nice.org.uk/guidance/ipg500/chapter/1-Recommendations.
12. Granquist EJ, et al. Outcomes and survivorship of Biomet microfixation total joint replacement system: results from an FDA Postmarket study. J Oral Maxillofac Surg. 2020;78(9):1499–508.
13. Johnson NR, et al. Total temporomandibular joint replacement prostheses: a systematic review and bias-adjusted meta-analysis. Int J Oral Maxillofac Surg. 2017;46(1):86–92.

14. Zou L, He D, Ellis E. A comparison of clinical follow-up of different Total temporomandibular joint replacement prostheses: a systematic review and meta-analysis. J Oral Maxillofac Surg. 2018;76(2):294–303.
15. Elledge R, et al. Review of emerging temporomandibular joint total joint replacement systems. Br J Oral Maxillofac Surg. 2019;57(8):722–8.
16. Mercuri LG, Caicedo MS. Material hypersensitivity and alloplastic temporomandibular joint replacement. J Oral Maxillofac Surg. 2019;77(7):1371–6.
17. Al-Kayat A, Bramley P. A modified pre-auricular approach to the temporomandibular joint and malar arch. Br J Oral Surg. 1979;17(2):91–103.
18. Wolford LM, Cardenas L. Idiopathic condylar resorption: diagnosis, treatment protocol, and outcomes. Am J Orthod Dentofacial Orthop. 1999;116(6):667–77.
19. Abrahamsson C, et al. Alterations of temporomandibular disorders before and after orthognathic surgery: a systematic review. Angle Orthod. 2007;77(4):729–34.
20. Al-Riyami S, Cunningham SJ, Moles DR. Orthognathic treatment and temporomandibular disorders: a systematic review. Part 2. Signs and symptoms and meta-analyses. Am J Orthod Dentofacial Orthop. 2009;136(5):626.e1-16, discussion 626–7.
21. Pruzansky S. Not all dwarfed mandibles are alike. Birth Defects Orig Artic Ser. 1969;1:120–9.
22. Kaban LB, Moses MH, Mulliken JB. Surgical correction of hemifacial microsomia in the growing child. Plast Reconstr Surg. 1988;82(1):9–19.
23. Saeed N, et al. Reconstruction of the temporomandibular joint autogenous compared with alloplastic. Br J Oral Maxillofac Surg. 2002;40(4):296–9.
24. Saeed NR, Kent JN. A retrospective study of the costochondral graft in TMJ reconstruction. Int J Oral Maxillofac Surg. 2003;32(6):606–9.
25. Keyser BR, et al. Alloplastic total temporomandibular joint replacement in skeletally immature patients: a pilot survey. Int J Oral Maxillofac Surg. 2020;49(9):1202–9.
26. McLoughlin PM, Hopper C, Bowley NB. Hyperplasia of the mandibular coronoid process: an analysis of 31 cases and a review of the literature. J Oral Maxillofac Surg. 1995;53(3):250–5.
27. Mulder CH, Kalaykova SI, Gortzak RA. Coronoid process hyperplasia: a systematic review of the literature from 1995. Int J Oral Maxillofac Surg. 2012;41(12):1483–9.
28. Padwa BL, et al. Pediatric chronic nonbacterial osteomyelitis of the jaw: clinical, radiographic, and histopathologic features. J Oral Maxillofac Surg. 2016;74(12):2393–402.
29. Gaal A, et al. Pediatric chronic nonbacterial osteomyelitis of the mandible: Seattle Children's hospital 22-patient experience. Pediatr Rheumatol Online J. 2020;18(1):4.

Temporomandibular Disorders: Case Histories

Stephen Davies and Emma Beecroft

1 Case History 1: Myofascial Pain

1.1 Patient's Aspiration

"I hope you can help with my pain, as it has been going on a long time and I find it very difficult to bear."

1.2 History of Presenting Complaint(s)

Site
"I feel it here, here and here".
Patient indicates, with their finger, temples and pre-auricular and cheek regions.
Onset/Event
"It just started about 5 years ago. There was no one thing that seemed to bring it on, although it was a very difficult time because I had started a new job and one of my parents was very ill."
Character of Pain and Severity
"It is an aching pain. It never really goes away. It varies between being a background ache to being a really bad pain that stops me from my normal activities. I just have to stop doing what I need to do, not that I can. I hope you can help me."
Associations

S. Davies (✉)
Division of Dentistry, University of Manchester, Manchester, UK
e-mail: stephen.j.davies@manchester.ac.uk

E. Beecroft
School of Dental Sciences, Newcastle University, Newcastle upon Tyne, UK
e-mail: emma.beecroft@newcastle.ac.uk

S. Davies et al. (eds.), *Temporomandibular Disorders in Primary Dental Care*,
BDJ Clinician's Guides, https://doi.org/10.1007/978-3-032-01301-9_7

"No, I can open my mouth normally. Although sometimes it does feel a bit tight and sore in my cheeks, when I try to open wide."

Timings

"Oh, it is nearly always worse in the mornings, when I wake up, and that is when it is stiff and sore. That is a real problem for me as I have a lot to do in the mornings. It is really gets me down."

Exacerbating/Relieving Factors

"Well, other than in the mornings, if I have had to do a lot of talking or hard chewing, it really sets it off. Just when I need it most, my jaw lets me down!"

"Yes, when I am tired the pain comes on."

"And when it is really cold outside."

"I noticed that it was much easier during a lovely holiday last year."

"I did try holding a hot water bottle against it when it was really bad, and it did help, but not for long. I only completed this the occasional day."

State of Mind or Mood

"Of course, I can't function normally, and I need to. It is really depressing to think I am going to live my life with this pain."

1.3 The Articulatory System Exam

Case 1 detailed articulatory exam is presented in Fig. 1. Note key findings of:

- Restricted interincisal opening at 33 mm under active stretch
- Familiar pain on palpation of masseter and temporalis bilaterally
- 2–3 mm slide from centric relation (CR) to centric occlusion (CO)
- Tongue scalloping and cheek ridging
- Positive pre-auricular pain ipsilateral to tongue spatula position on compression testing suggesting myogenous origin (Fig. 1)

1.4 Further Investigations

This individual mentioned a number of psychosocial points in their history which warrant further investigation as per axis II of the DC/TMD [1]. Socially, the individual reported a "difficult time" when starting a new job and an unwell family member at the approximate time of onset of symptoms. Further exploration of these factors is important, if the issues are still ongoing and the individual's ability to cope is affected, and such factors can heavily influence the course of their condition.

When questioned further, the individual reported their new job has actually become a positive factor and they are well settled and found the working environment supportive, and so this needed no further consideration in terms of management strategies. Conversely, the individual had now become primary carer for their unwell parent, in addition to the pre-existing responsibilities of two dependent teenage children and full-time employment. When questioned further, the individual reported feeling "overwhelmed" and no longer had time to "even do my Pilates classes".

Exploration around sleep was appropriate due to the report of tiredness being an exacerbating feature. The individual reported they had no issues getting or staying asleep but explained that they were in a habit of staying up very late to "get everything done".

Triggers for more detailed psychological assessment were clear with the individual expressing her condition was both "difficult to bear" and the concept

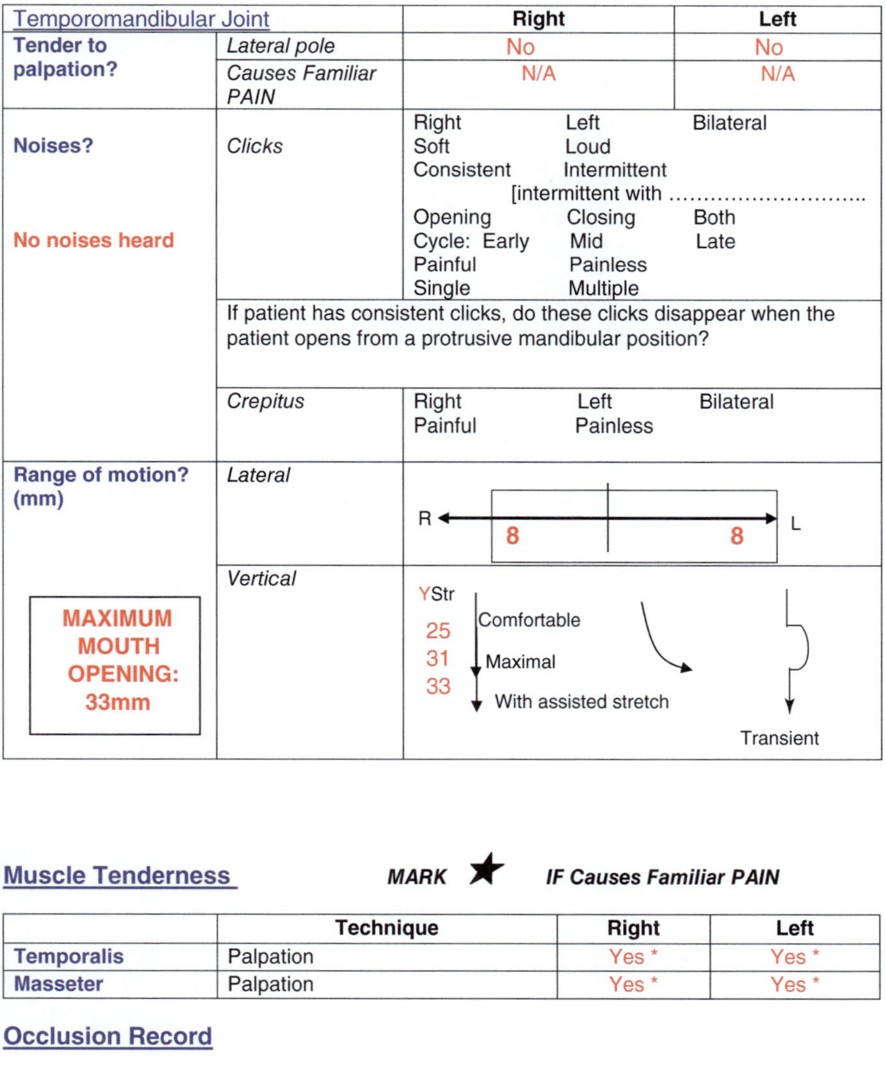

Temporomandibular Joint		Right	Left
Tender to palpation?	*Lateral pole*	No	No
	Causes Familiar PAIN	N/A	N/A
Noises? **No noises heard**	*Clicks*	Right Left Bilateral Soft Loud Consistent Intermittent [intermittent with .... Opening Closing Both Cycle: Early Mid Late Painful Painless Single Multiple	
	If patient has consistent clicks, do these clicks disappear when the patient opens from a protrusive mandibular position?		
	Crepitus	Right Left Bilateral Painful Painless	
Range of motion? (mm)	*Lateral*	R 8 8 L	
MAXIMUM MOUTH OPENING: 33mm	*Vertical*	YStr 25 Comfortable 31 Maximal 33 With assisted stretch Transient	

Muscle Tenderness ***MARK ★ IF Causes Familiar PAIN***

	Technique	Right	Left
Temporalis	Palpation	Yes *	Yes *
Masseter	Palpation	Yes *	Yes *

Occlusion Record

Fig. 1 Case 1, myofascial pain detailed articulatory examination

Skeletal	Class I		
Angles	Class I		
Static occlusion	Does C.O occur in C.R? No		
	If not – premature contact in C.R? *Roughly:* *Consistent Left 1st Premolar region* *or* *Exactly:* *Not recorded at this time* *Direction of slide from C.R to C.O:* 2-3 mm, to right and anterior *Freedom in centric occlusion?* yes		
Dynamic occlusion		**Right**	**Left**
	Non-working side interferences?	No	No
	Working side interferences?	No	No
	Crossover position: *Non-working side*	–	–
	Working side	-	-
	Canine guidance?	Yes	yes
	Group function?	-	-

Excessive wear X *Evidence of tooth/restoration fracture* X

Cheek ridging *yes* *tongue scalloping* *yes*

Compression Test *Tongue Spatulae*	**Elicits Pain?** Pain on RHS?	Pain on LHS?
on RHS	☐Yes *myogenic*	☐No *arthrogenic*
on LHS	☐ No *arthrogenic*	☐ Yes *myogenic*

Fig. 1 (continued)

of continued pain was "depressing". In this case, both the FLATS screening tool, outlined in Chapter "Psychological Considerations", and for formative assessment of symptoms of anxiety and depression, the patient health questionnaire 4 (PHQ 4) score were calculated using a freely available tool from the Royal College of Surgeons' Faculty of Dental Practitioners at this web address [2]. PHQ-4 consists of four questions which assess symptoms of anxiety and depression and are routinely used by medical colleagues supporting care transition if required. This patient scored 1 point on FLATS, supporting shortened review periods, and reassuringly 3 points on PHQ4 indicating mild symptoms of anxiety and depression only.

1.5 Diagnosis

- Broad group diagnosis: myogenous TMD (M-TMD)
- Specific TMD sub-classification: myofascial pain affecting bilateral masseters and temporalis

1.6 Compounding Factors Specific to This Case

- Weight of familial responsibility
- Inadequate sleep
- Cessation of enjoyment activities (Pilates)
- Mild symptoms of anxiety and depression

1.7 Management

1.7.1 Explanation and Supported Self-Management

- Findings were discussed with the patient collaboratively, listening carefully to their ideas, concerns and expectations [ICE] and allowing time for questions and clarifications.
- Patient was provided with a diagnosis at first consultation. It was carefully explained that although very painful, significant improvement can be expected with consistent self-management. Explanation of diagnosis was provided in detail (see Chapter "Management", for examples of this).
- Expectations were managed. It was explained that the patient needs to play an active role in self-management, including strategies targeted to ease pain around the jaw and face. The patient was advised to focus on management rather than elimination of pain.
- The individual was signposted to appropriate support resources, and it was advised that these resources be shared with friends and family to help them understand the individual's condition.
- Support resources specific to this case were:
  - Management of painful temporomandibular disorder in adults NHS England Getting It Right First Time (GIRFT) and Royal College of Surgeons' Faculty of Dental Surgery Patient Summary Document, which includes both further information and reassurance with regard to the condition, and active self-management strategy details likely to be beneficial [3].
  - Explanation on how sleep can affect the experience of pain and sleep hygiene resources. (Refer to Chapter "Psychological Considerations" for more detail.)
  - Due to pain on eating hard foods being an issue, they were directed to the temporomandibular joint associations "TMD, nutrition and you" guide which supports diet modification to reduce pain whilst capitalising on nutrition [4].
- The individual's current mild symptom score of depression and anxiety was openly discussed, and an explanation as to how their heavy social burden, mood and pain can all interplay was provided. The individual felt they would not benefit from further medical assessment with regard to their psychosocial status, and so a broader focus on more holistic factors known to influence pain overall was

advised. Specific to this patient, we discussed ensuring adequate time to care for themselves as well as others and re-engagement with activities which provided escape and joy (Pilates) as initial strategies.

1.8 Muscle Therapy

The patient was provided with the NHS England Getting It Right First Time (GIRFT) and Royal College of Surgeons' Faculty of Dental Surgery supported QR code which directs the patient to videos of muscular therapy techniques for use at home (Fig. 2) [3].

- The patient was complemented on their use of hot water bottles, and it was reinformed that twice daily heat application for up to 20 min, when performed regularly rather than intermittently, would likely have a more positive beneficial effect. The patient was advised in addition to complete facial massage of the masseter and temporalis twice daily.
- Self-physiotherapy in the form of N-Stretch and static stretch exercises to improve coordination and increase mandibular opening, respectively, were advised and demonstrated. Box 1 outlines these exercises in detail.

Box 1: N-Stretch and Static-Stretch Exercises

N Stretch jaw Exercise: Advise the patient to open normally and then curl their tongue to the roof of their mouth with the tip of the tongue pointing towards the soft palate. Reassure them that they feel their lower jaw move backwards slightly. Keeping your tongue in this position advise the individual to close in a slow controlled manner over five-six seconds (one set) and to complete 20 repetitions up to four times a day.

Static-Stretch Exercise: The individual was advised directly after applying heat to the facial muscles to then gently open as far as is comfortable. At that point they should place their index fingers on the lower canine teeth and your thumbs on your upper canine teeth (fingers and thumbs will be crossed) and stretch gently for 30 seconds to the point of discomfort and a small amount further and hold for 30 seconds. This should be gently repeated 5-6 times 2-3 times daily.

Fig. 2 NHS England and Royal College of Surgeons Faculty of Dental Surgery supported patient video QR code which directs patients to TMD advice, self-physiotherapy, jaw exercise, thermal modalities and facial massage videos to enhance supported self-management

1.9 Occlusal Therapy

There may be a case for a stabilisation splint, due to the CR to CO slide, but consideration of this was decided to be made at a 6–8-week review appointment forming part of an adjunctive treatment plan.

1.9.1 Outcome

The patient attended happy and grateful at 6–8-week review appointment. They have reignited their social life, spending time with friends socially. After discussing their condition with their family, a chore rota helped distribute home care tasks, and their teenage children were supportive with this. The patient had engaged positively with heat application, facial massage and jaw exercises. Adding a short lunchtime walk and 2 Pilates classes a week had supported mood, and the patient reported they were more tired due to gentle increase in exercise and so were sleeping much better. The cyclical nature of the condition was discussed to ensure this would not demotivate the patient should pain start to increase once more.

2 Case History 2: Disc Displacement with Reduction

2.1 Patient's Aspiration

"I hope that you can stop the constant clicking of my jaw."

2.2 History of Presenting Complaint(S)

Site
"In front of my left ear."
Onset/Event
"I have always had a clicky jaw, which tended to come and go. I have noticed that the click is a bit louder over the last 6 months."
Character of Pain and Severity
"I don't feel any real pain. It is the noise I am concerned about. I am worried that it could be arthritis."
Associations/Timings
"Slight discomfort only after a lot of chewing or talking."
Timings
"I hear a click, every time I open my mouth."
"I am always able to open and close normally. It never gets stuck."
Exacerbating/Relieving Factors

"It's just there, nothing makes it better or worse."

State of Mind or Mood

"It doesn't get me down. It can be a bit embarrassing socially, but my family have got used to my clicking jaw! If you are going to tell me that it is something serious, then I expect that I will feel differently."

2.3 The Articulatory System Exam

Case 2 detailed articulatory exam is presented in Fig. 3. Note key findings of:

- Consistent left TMJ single click
- Click painless
- Click in mid-1/3 of opening cycle
- Corrected deviation of mandible at point of click
- No restricted opening
- No pain when palpating TMJ or muscles of mastication

2.4 Further Investigations

Nil

2.5 Diagnosis

- Broad group diagnosis: arthrogenous TMD (A-TMD)
- Specific TMD sub-classification: left-sided pain free disc displacement with reduction

2.6 Management

1. Explanation of the functional anatomy of a TMJ and of the mechanics of DDwR.
2. Reassure that this is not a serious condition; in fact, this is a "noisy version of normal".
3. Reassure that the noise is NOT arthritis and does not indicate damage to the joint.
4. Discuss disc displacements have a good prognosis and generally remain stable rather than progress [5].
5. Discuss the discs ability to change shape over time and that clicks can get more of less noisy and this is entirely normal.
6. Advise no management can guarantee to eliminate click, and discuss how no active management is required in this case.
5. Advise the benefit of a mouth prop for anything other than the shortest of dental visits to support the temporomandibular joint apparatus.

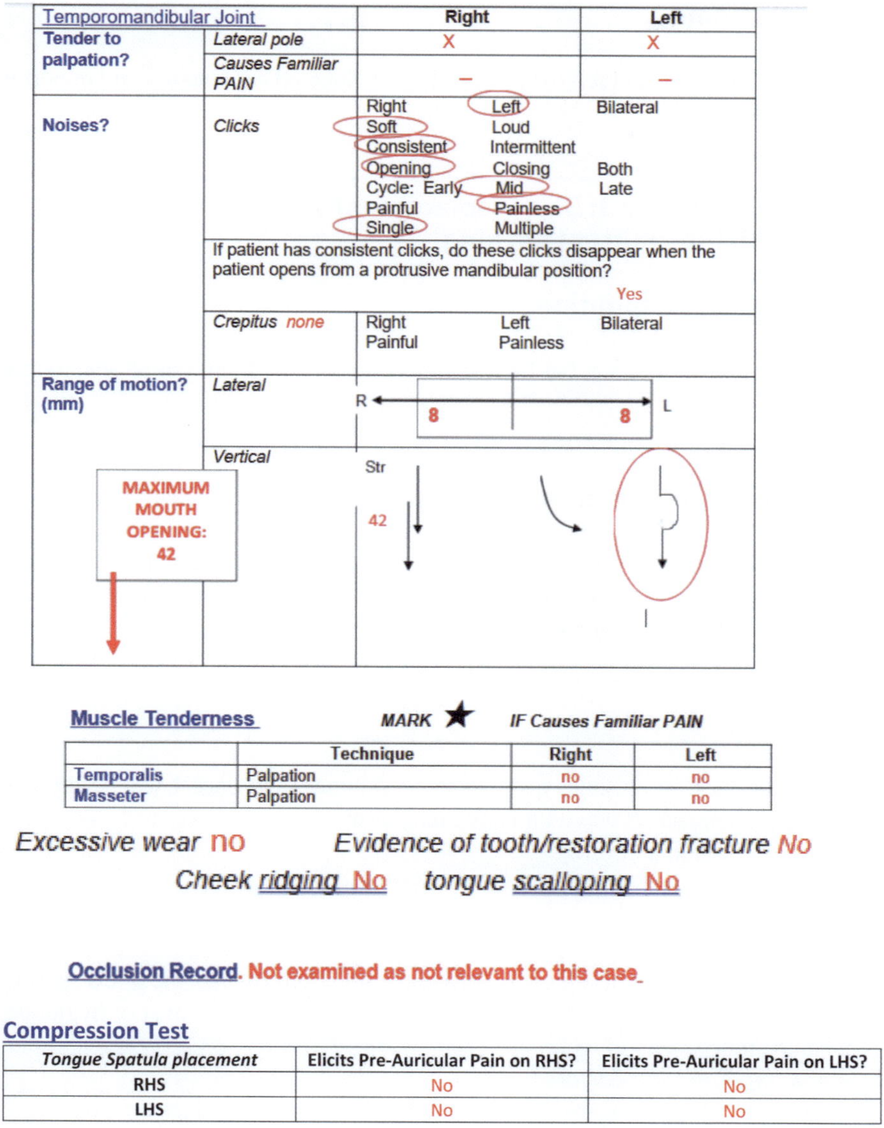

Temporomandibular Joint		Right	Left
Tender to palpation?	Lateral pole	X	X
	Causes Familiar PAIN	–	–
Noises?	Clicks	Right / **(Left)** / Bilateral **(Soft)** / Loud **(Consistent)** / Intermittent **(Opening)** / Closing / Both Cycle: Early / **(Mid)** / Late Painful / **(Painless)** **(Single)** / Multiple	
	If patient has consistent clicks, do these clicks disappear when the patient opens from a protrusive mandibular position? Yes		
	Crepitus none	Right / Left / Bilateral Painful / Painless	
Range of motion? (mm)	Lateral	R 8 – 8 L	
MAXIMUM MOUTH OPENING: 42	Vertical	Str 42	

Muscle Tenderness MARK ★ IF Causes Familiar PAIN

	Technique	Right	Left
Temporalis	Palpation	no	no
Masseter	Palpation	no	no

Excessive wear no Evidence of tooth/restoration fracture No

Cheek ridging No tongue scalloping No

Occlusion Record. Not examined as not relevant to this case

Compression Test

Tongue Spatula placement	Elicits Pre-Auricular Pain on RHS?	Elicits Pre-Auricular Pain on LHS?
RHS	No	No
LHS	No	No

Fig. 3 Case 2, disc displacement with reduction detailed articulatory examination

2.7 Outcome

Patient was reassured and felt happy after having detailed explanation and opportunity to discuss.

3 Case History 3: Disc Displacement with Reduction with Intermittent Locking

3.1 Patient's Aspiration

"I can live with the clicking, but I am anxious that one day I will not be able to free the lock and open normally."

3.2 History of Presenting Complaint(s)

"I have had a click from my left jaw joint for years, but about 5 years ago, it has been locking, so I can't open properly. It releases with a big click after I wiggle it about a bit. The locking happens about 3 times a week."

Site
"In front of my left ear."
Onset/Event
"Each of the locking episodes lasts about 15 minutes, and once I wiggle my jaw enough, it releases. It was a bit frightening at first."
Character of Pain and Severity
"I don't feel any pain when it is clicking, but when I can't open my mouth, it can be a bit uncomfortable."
Associations/Timings
"It can be worse in the mornings, when I wake up. Then it takes me a few goes to get it working properly again. Also, after a long visit to the dentist or hygienist, it can be more likely to lock."
Exacerbating/Relieving Factors
"If I try to relax my jaw, it seems easier to unlock it. Panicking does not help!"
State of Mind or Mood
"No, it doesn't get me down, but I might feel differently depending what you tell me."

3.3 The Articulatory System Exam

Case 3 detailed articulatory exam is presented in Fig. 4.

Note the key findings:

- Painless left-sided consistent click late in opening cycle
- Protrusion to class III incisor relationship eliminated click
- No pain in muscles of mastication
- Lasting deviation to the LHS during opening
- Reduced interincisal opening 32 mm when lock present, 40 mm when lock freed
- Restricted right lateral excursion

Temporomandibular Joint		Right	Left
Tender to palpation?	*Lateral pole*	No	No
	Causes Familiar PAIN	**N/A**	N/A
Noises?	*When Clicking*	Right Left Bilateral Soft Loud Consistent Intermittent [intermittent with .... Opening Closing Both Cycle: Early Mid Late Painful Painless Single Multiple	
	If patient has consistent clicks, do these clicks disappear when the patient opens from a protrusive mandibular position? Only with mandible in a Cl III incisor relationship		
	Crepitus *none*	Right Left Bilateral Painful Painless	
Range of motion? (mm) **MAXIMUM MOUTH OPENING:** **32 with lock, 40mm when lock freed**	*Lateral*	R ← → L **8** clicking **4** locked **8**	
	Vertical click occurred at 32 mm, then able to open to 40mm	locked. clicking	

Muscle Tenderness *MARK* ★ *IF Causes Familiar PAIN*

	Technique	Right	Left
Temporalis	Palpation	No	No
Masseter	Palpation	No	No

Occlusion Record. **Not examined as not relevant in this case**

Fig. 4 Case 3, disc displacement with reduction with intermittent locking detailed articulatory examination

3.4 Further Investigations

Nil

3.5 Diagnosis

- Broad group diagnosis: arthrogenous TMD (A-TMD)
- Specific TMD sub-classification: disc displacement with reduction (DDwR) with intermittent locking (essentially an intermittent and very-short-lived event of a disc displacement without reduction)

3.6 Management

1. Reassurance that this is not a serious condition and that given how long it has been present, it is unlikely to become permanently locked.
2. Explanation of the functional anatomy of a TMJ, and of the mechanics of DDwR, and of DDwR with intermittent locking.
3. Patient was shown the correct unlocking manoeuvres to utilise at home to give them the best chance of early reduction, should a lock present.
4. Advise that the patient is provided with a mouth prop for dental treatment of any substantial length.

3.6.1 Outcome

The patient felt happy that the lock was something it was safe to live with. They were happy to continue to unlock themselves once they were advised their "wiggling" to reduce the jaw would not cause any damage over time.

4 Case History 4: Subluxation

4.1 Patient's Aspiration

"I would like to know why my jaw keeps clunking. I am worried that it might be serious.

It is just the clunking feeling. I can always open ok."

4.2 History of Presenting Complaint(s)

Site
"In front of my left ear."
Onset/Event
"It started about 5 years ago, when I yawned, and heard a big click on this jaw joint. The jaw got stuck open for a few seconds, I wiggle it, and it closed again."
Character of Pain and Severity
"I don't feel any pain, but when it gets stuck open, it is annoying."
Associations/Timings
"Ever since that first clunk, when I open wide, there is a massive clunk."
Exacerbating/Relieving Factors
"The only way I can avoid it is to not open so wide."
State of Mind or Mood
"No, it doesn't get me down."

4.3 The Articulatory System Exam

Case 4 detailed articulatory exam is presented in Fig. 5.

Note key findings:

- TMJ single painless click that occurs at extreme opening.
- With noise, the jaw can lock open for a few seconds; self-movement allows normal position to resume.
- No pain when palpating TMJ or muscles of mastication.

4.4 Further Investigations

Nil

4.5 Diagnosis

- Broad group diagnosis: arthrogenous TMD (A-TMD)
- Specific TMD sub-classification: subluxation

4.6 Management

1. Explanation of functional anatomy of TMJ.
2. Suggest avoidance of extremes of opening which is trigger for subluxation in this case.

Temporomandibular Joint		Right	Left
Tender to palpation?	*Lateral pole*	No	No
	Causes Familiar PAIN	**N/A**	N/A
Noises?	*Clicks*	Right ~~Left~~ Bilateral Soft Loud Consistent ~~Intermittent~~ [intermittent with .... Opening Closing ~~Both~~ Cycle: Early ~~Mid~~ Late Painful Painless Single ~~Multiple~~	
	If patient has consi~~stent clic~~ks, do these clicks disappear when the patient opens from a protrusive mandibular position?		
	Crepitus	Right Left Bilateral Painful Painless	
Range of motion? (mm)	*Lateral*	R ← **10** | **10** → L	
	Vertical	45 ↓	

Muscle Tenderness

MARK ★ ***IF Causes Familiar PAIN***

	Technique	Right	Left
Temporalis	Palpation	No	No
Masseter	Palpation	No	No

Occlusion Record. Not Recorded as not relevant

Fig. 5 Case history 4, subluxation detailed articulatory examination

3. Reassure benign nature and stress jaw is not being damaged; reassure positive long-term prognosis.
   - Advised to complete isometric tension jaw exercises to strengethen jaw muscles, this may help resist subluxation.
4. Advice mouth prop to support opening, at less than maximum, during all dental visits.
5. Surgical intervention is only considered when a patient is suffering from repeated, frequent and lengthy episodes of open lock that require clinician led reduction.

5 Case History 5: Repeated TMJ Luxation (Dislocation)

5.1 Patient's Aspiration

"I am desperate to stop my jaw from dislocating. It happened twice last month."

5.2 History of Presenting Complaint

Site
"It seems to be both jaw joints."
Onset
"It started about 3 years ago, completely out of the blue. I opened my mouth wide, and I just could not close it."
Pain
"Yes, it is painful when my mouth is stuck open."
Associations
"It happens when I open wide to eat a large portion of food, or when I yawn."
"Visits to the dentists are very difficult for us both."
Timings
"Since then it has happened about every two months. Sometimes I can push it back, but usually I have to the hospital, for them to force it back closed and each time I have to go off to A&E for them to put it back, usually under sedation."
State of Mind or Mood
"I am worn out by this, not just because of when it happens it is horrible but the anxiety I feel when eating, or feel a yawn coming on."

5.3 The Articulatory System Exam

Examination was restricted due to patient anxiety; muscles of mastication did not elicit pain. Patient was fearful to open wider than 25 mm due to fear of dislocation; however, the patient history itself is diagnostic of luxation (dislocation) of the temporomandibular joint.

5.4 Further Investigations

Nil

5.5 Diagnosis

- Broad group diagnosis: arthrogenous TMD (A-TMD)
- Specific TMD sub-classification: Luxation (TMJ dislocation)

5.6 Management

1. Explanation.
2. Advise to continue with avoidance and supporting any yawn with the back of the hand placed gently under chin to support jaw and limit its opening during a yawn.
3. Advise immediately after luxation to try applying warm compresses to the pre-auricular regions as an aid to muscle relaxation prior to attempting self-reduction.
4. Advise on the use of a small mouth prop to support the TMJ and limit risk of luxation in the dental setting.
5. Referral to an oral and maxillofacial unit for assessment to identify if any underlying predisposing factors present and whether surgical intervention would be indicated given the number of dislocations.

5.6.1 Outcome

The maxillofacial team found that there was a very shallow articular eminence on the right side, which the condylar head moved over easily. The left side however had a very acute eminence, which meant that once the condylar head moved over this, it could not easily reduce. An eminectomy was completed on the left side under general anaesthesia. Following surgery, the condylar head bilaterally was able to relocate easily back into the articular fossa. This meant that the dislocations no longer required interventive treatment to relocate. The patient needed no further acute emergency department attendances and was very happy with the result.

6 Case History 6: Limited Opening Due to Muscular Guarding

6.1 Patient's Aspiration

"I hope you can help, I cannot open my jaw fully and it is also painful in my face sometimes".

6.2 History of Present Complaint

Site

"I feel it here, here…." Patient indicates, with their finger and their cheek regions.

Onset/Event

"I can't really remember when this started. To some extent, I think it has been present for ages. I sometimes feel that my mouth will not open as wide as it should, and when I try, it hurts here [indicated cheeks]."

Character of Pain and Severity

"It is not really serious pain. In fact, sometimes, it is not there at all. It is definitely worse in the mornings when I wake up. Sometimes, it is difficult to get the spoon in my mouth for breakfast."

"The worse time is a visit to the dentist or hygienist."

Associations

"It is worse when I am tired or stressed. The last few years have been difficult."

"I find myself with my teeth locked together during the day."

State of Mind or Mood

"No, it doesn't get me down, although a friend told me he thought it might be that my jaw joints were beginning to seize up. That is a bit worrying, I had an aunt who had terrible Rheumatoid Arthritis".

6.3 The Articulatory System Exam

Case 6 detailed articulatory exam is presented in Fig. 6.

Note the key findings:

- No indication that there is any problem within the joints.
- Palpation of enlarged masseter muscles was tender and elicited a familiar pain.
- Passive stretch increases interincisal opening from 31 to 39 mm.
- Clinician notes that passive stretch of the muscles increases interincisal opening and feels soft (soft end point).

6.4 Further Investigations

Nil

6.5 Diagnosis

- Broad group diagnosis: myogenous TMD (M-TMD).
- Specific TMD sub-classification: myofascial pain with trismus secondary to muscular guarding.

6.6 Management

1. Findings were discussed with the patient collaboratively, listening carefully to their ideas, concerns and expectations and allowing time for questions and clarifications.
2. Patient was provided with a diagnosis of myogenous TMD at first consultation and explanation on how clenching can enlarge and shorten the masseter muscles [it is an isometric exercise].

Temporomandibular Joint		Right	Left
Tender to palpation?	*Lateral pole*	No	No
	Causes Familiar PAIN	**N/A**	N/A
Noises? **No noises heard**	*Clicks*	Right Left Bilateral Soft Loud Consistent Intermittent [intermittent with .... Opening Closing Both Cycle: Early Mid Late Painful Painless Single Multiple	
	If patient has consistent clicks, do these clicks disappear when the patient opens from a protrusive mandibular position?		
	Crepitus	Right Left Bilateral Painful Painless	
Range of motion? (mm) **MAXIMUM MOUTH OPENING: 39mm soft end point**	*Lateral*	R ← 8 | 8 → L	
	Vertical	Str 18 Comfortable 28 Maximal 39 With assisted stretch Transient	

Muscle Tenderness

MARK ★ IF Causes Familiar PAIN

	Technique	Right	Left
Temporalis	Palpation	Yes	Yes
Masseter	Palpation	Yes ★ Felt enlarged	Yes ★ Felt enlarged

Occlusion Record. No indication for doing an Occlusal Examinatin

Excessive wear X *Evidence of tooth/restoration fracture* X

Cheek ridging yes *tongue scalloping* yes

Compression Test

Tongue Spatulae

Elicits Pain?

	Pain on RHS?	Pain on LHS?
on RHS	☐ Yes *myogenic*	☐ No *arthrogenic*
on LHS	☐ No *arthrogenic*	☐ Yes *myogenic*

Fig. 6 Case 6, limited opening due to muscular guarding detailed articulatory examination

3. Reassurance that there is no indication of joint pathology and it is not arthritis.
4. Explanation of diagnosis was provided in detail (see Chapter "Management").
5. Advised to use warm compresses in cheek regions [TDS for several weeks: "It is treatment not just pain relief"].
6. Shown technique for passive stretching and advised to complete twice daily, ideally after warm compresses.
7. Referral for physiotherapy.
8. Advice GDP to always provide patient with benefit of a mouth prop other than for the shortest of visits.
9. Following review stabilisation splint may be appropriate adjunctive management strategy.

6.6.1 Outcome

Passive stretching twice daily at home meant that unassisted mouth opening at review appointment had increased to 42 mm; and conservative strategies had resulced muscular discomfort the patient was extremely happy.

7 Case 7: Myofascial Pain Post-orthodontic Treatment

7.1 Patient's Aspiration

"Eliminate pain."

7.2 History of Presenting Complaint(s)

Site:
Pain in their left cheek and in front of the left ear.
Onset/Event
The pain reportedly started shortly after completion of orthodontic treatment 3 years ago; this, also, coincided with a stressful time.
Character of Pain and Severity
Ache varying between 4 and 7 out of 10.
*Associations/*Timings
There is a feeling of a variable restriction in mouth opening.
Timings
Pain is constantly present.
Exacerbating/Relieving Factors
It is worse in the morning and after jaw use.
Painkillers, such as paracetamol, can help for short periods when pain is really problematic.
State of Mind or Mood
Ongoing pain has influenced the individual's mood, which at times can be low.

7.3 The Articulatory System Exam (See Fig. 7)

Key findings of articulatory examination listed below:

- The lateral poles of both TMJs were *not* sensitive to palpation.
- Comfortable interincisal opening = 16 mm and straight.
- Unassisted interincisal opening = 33 mm; increased to 35 mm with passive stretching.

Temporomandibular Joint		Right	Left
Tender to palpation?	*Lateral pole*	No	No
	Causes Familiar PAIN	**N/A**	N/A
Noises? **No noises heard**	*Clicks*	Right Left Bilateral Soft Loud Consistent Intermittent [intermittent with .... Opening Closing Both Cycle: Early Mid Late Painful Painless Single Multiple	
	If patient has consistent clicks, do these clicks disappear when the patient opens from a protrusive mandibular position?		
	Crepitus	Right Left Bilateral Painful Painless	
Range of motion? (mm)	*Lateral*	R ← 7 | 7 → L	
MAXIMUM MOUTH OPENING: 35mm	*Vertical*	Str (circled) 16 Comfortable 33 Maximal 35 With assisted stretching	

Muscle Tenderness *MARK* ★ *IF Causes Familiar PAIN*

	Technique	Right	Left
Temporalis	Palpation	Yes ★	Yes ★
Masseter	Palpation	Yes ★	Yes ★

Fig. 7 Case 7, myofascial pain post orthodontic care detailed articulatory examination

Occlusion Record. This examination only needs to be done if some form of splint therapy might be considered

Skeletal	Class I		
Angles	Class I		
	Does C.O occur in C.R? No difficult to find because of muscle bracing		
	If not – premature contact in C.R? *Roughly:* *Consistent right 1st Premolar region* *or* *Exactly:* *Not recorded at this time* *Direction of slide from C.R to C.O:* 3 mm, to left and vertical *Freedom in centric occlusion?* yes		
Dynamic occlusion		**Right**	**Left**
	Non-working side interferences?	Yes	Yes
	Working side interferences?	No	No
	Crossover position: *Non-working side*	–	–
	Working side	-	-
	Canine guidance?	Yes	yes
	Group function?	-	-

Excessive wear X *Evidence of tooth/restoration fracture* X

Cheek ridging X *tongue scalloping* yes

Compression Test

Tongue Spatulae

Elicits Pre-Auricular Pain?

	Pain on RHS?	**Pain on LHS?**
on RHS	☐ **Yes** *myogenic*	☐ No *arthrogenic*
on LHS	☐ No *arthrogenic*	☐ Yes *myogenic*

Fig. 7 (continued)

- All muscles were very tender to palpation and elicited familiar pain.
- A consistent premature contact was identified in centric relation (CR); it was in the right-hand-side premolar region.
- From this premature contact in CR, there was a slide to centric occlusion. The slide was about 3 mm, vertical and to the left.

- There was Freedom in CO.
- There were posterior interferences on the non-working sides.
- Marked tongue scalloping, but no cheek ridging was noted.
- Compression test was indicative of myogenous pain.

7.4 Further Investigations

The patient's history presented several psychosocial factors which require further investigation. Onset was reported at a stressful time. The patient's current stress levels, coping and support strategies need discussing. The patient reports when questioned that they have been going through a stressful period of work and additionally their relationship with their partner has been difficult. They report they have thought about looking for a new job to see if another environment may help them.

The individual also stated that their mood can sometimes be "low". When you discuss this further with them, you are the first health professional they have disclosed this to. You complete the PHQ 4 screener, and they score 8 indicating evidence of moderate psychosocial distress. You openly discuss this with the patient who, though well supported by family and friends and safe, does feel further support may be beneficial as they have felt low for a little while now. You write a referral letter to the patient's general medical practitioner outlining the patient's symptoms and PHQ 4 score requesting they formally assess, diagnose and offer management as they see fit for potential comorbid mental health issues.

7.5 Diagnosis

- Broad group diagnosis: myogenous TMD (M-TMD)
- Specific TMD sub-classification: myofascial pain

7.6 Other Potential Important Features of this Case

1. Muscular guarding

   Likely the cause of intermittent restricted opening. Management strategies as outlined in case 6 need to be initiated.
2. Potential for comorbid depression (discussed further below)
3. Orthodontic treatment

There seems to be is temporal relationship between the onset of this muscular discomfort and the completion of the orthodontic treatment, although there were other factors in place at the same time (stress). The orthodontic result is good. It is unusual for there to be a lasting discomfort associated with the provision of the occlusal change via the orthodontic treatment. The onset of this discomfort is not a contra-indication to the provision of orthodontic treatment, in the way that a pre-existing temporomandibular disorder may have been. It is not surprising that some patients may experience mild discomfort whilst they adapt to the new occlusion and jaw relationship that some orthodontic treatment provides. It should, however, be stressed that in the majority of patients, this is a short-term consequence. The possibility of it happening is not a reason for avoiding orthodontic treatment, which will have long-term benefit to the patient. If any management of this short-term discomfort is needed, it will entail reassurance as part of supported self-management, together with treatment directed towards the muscles, for example, warm compresses. It is, however, advisable that an initial orthodontic examination should include the discovery of any pre-existing TMD.

7.7 Management

7.7.1 Explanation and Reassurance

Detailed discussions around cause of pain, the patient's diagnosis and why pain in this region can be so impactful should be provided to educate and reassure the patient. Education as to why both stress and periods of low mood are likely to have a bidirectional relationship with pain should be provided. Though they do not cause pain, their presence will impact how the pain is felt, and management of pain must involve both mitigation of stress and support with mood where possible.

In addition to acting as an ear to listen and referring the patient to their general medical practitioner, it would be advisable to discuss how they might to seek some help in reducing the effects of their stress and mood by identifying effective coping strategies, and these could include continuing to engage in social activities, to take time every day to complete an activity which brings them joy, using breathing practices to manage stress and ensuring they take gentle exercise daily.

7.7.2 Expectation Management

The patient was specifically requesting elimination of their pain. Honest discussions should be provided to manage the patient's expectations. Discussion as to the fact there is no "cure for TMD" should be provided. Advise that working towards management rather than cure is a realistic aim.

7.7.3 Supported Self-Management

This patient was provided with links to the Royal College of Surgeons' QR code for supported self-management videos (Fig. 2), alongside the RCS patient support document. They were advised to complete jaw exercises as outlined in Fig. 3, in addition to warm compresses and facial massage targeting the masseters bilaterally, all of which should be advised twice a day for 6 weeks.

7.7.4 Adjunctive Management

On review, which should be completed 6–8 weeks after initial consultation, if there has not been a significant improvement with the supported self-management, adjunctive management strategies can be discussed, and in a process of shared decision-making with the individual, next steps can be determined.

Case-specific adjunctive management strategies:

2a. *Splint therapy.* Consideration could be given to some form of splint therapy, as additional management. Whilst a splint is not direct treatment to the muscles, it may act as an aid to muscle recovery.
2b. *Physiotherapy.* Referral for formal physiotherapy could be discussed to capitalize on management of myogenous TMD.
2c. *Acupuncture.* Referral for acupuncture to affected musculature has been shown to support pain management.

8 Case History 8: Myofascial Pain After a Single Extraction

8.1 Patient's Aspiration

"I don't know how I should fit my teeth together."

8.2 History of Presenting Complaint(s)

Onset/Event

"This happened after I had a tooth extracted [upper left second premolar] 2 months ago."

Character of Pain and Severity

"I am also suffering pain in my face. There is always an ache which sometimes becomes very intense."

Site:

"It is down the side of my face."

Associations

"I find that my lower jaw does not sit right against my upper jaw, and I keep moving it to try and find the right position."

Timings

"I never had any of these problems until I had that tooth out."

Exacerbating/Relieving Factors

"I can have difficulty in speaking."

"Fortunately, I sleep very well, and always feels rested when I wake up."

State of Mind or Mood

"I am finding it annoying not being able to find my correct bite."

8.3 The Articulatory System Exam

Case 8 detailed articulatory exam is presented in Fig. 8. Note the key findings of:

- Familiar pain bilateral masseters and temporalis
- Premature contact in centric relation
- No consistent nor balanced centric occlusion
- Compression test positive for myogenous pain bilaterally

8.4 Further Investigations

Nil

Temporomandibular Joint		Right	Left
Tender to palpation?	*Lateral pole*	slight	slight
	Causes Familiar PAIN	**No**	NO
Noises? **No noises heard**	*Clicks*	Right Left Bilateral Soft Loud Consistent Intermittent [intermittent with .... Opening Closing Both Cycle: Early Mid Late Painful Painless Single Multiple	
	If patient has consistent clicks, do these clicks disappear when the patient opens from a protrusive mandibular position?		
	Crepitus	Right Left Bilateral Painful Painless	
Range of motion? (mm)	*Lateral*	R ← **8** | **9** → L	
MAXIMUM MOUTH OPENING: 39mm	*Vertical*	Str (circled) 19 Comfortable 33 Maximal 39 With assisted stretch	

Muscle Tenderness ***MARK*** ★ ***IF Causes Familiar PAIN***

	Technique	Right	Left
Temporalis	Palpation	Yes ★	Yes ★
Masseter	Palpation	Yes ★	Yes ★

Occlusion Record

Fig. 8 Case 8, onset of symptoms after single extraction detailed articulatory examination

Static occlusion **Centric Occlusion is not balanced** **There is no contact between the 2nd molars on the LHS**	Does C.O occur in C.R? No		
	If not – premature contact in C.R? *Roughly:* *Consistent Left 1st Premolar region* *or* *Exactly Mesial facing incline of palatal cusp of Upper left 1st premolar against distal facing incline of lower left canine* *Direction of slide from C.R to C.O:* patient does not slide from the Premature Contact in CR to a *consistent CO* *Freedom in centric occlusion?* *Yes*		
Dynamic occlusion		**Right**	**Left**
	Non-working side interferences?	yes	yes
	Working side interferences?	No	No
	Crossover position: *Non-working side*	–	–
	Working side	-	-
	Canine guidance?	Yes	yes
	Group function?	-	-

Excessive wear X *Evidence of tooth/restoration fracture* X

Cheek ridging yes *tongue scalloping* yes

Compression Test ***Tongue Spatulae***	**Elicits Pre-Auricular Pain?**	
	Pain on RHS?	**Pain on LHS?**
on RHS	☐**YES** *myogenic*	☐No *arthrogenic*
on LHS	☐ No *arthrogenic*	☐ YES *myogenic*

Fig. 8 (continued)

8.5 Diagnosis

- Broad group diagnosis: myogenous TMD (M-TMD)
- Specific TMD sub-classification: myofascial pain affecting masseter and temporalis muscles

8.6 Other Features of This Case

In this case, the onset of symptoms coincided with the extraction of a single tooth after which the patient reported a change in her occlusion. This close temporal relationship between the signs and symptoms of myofascial pain and the perceived change in occlusion suggest that *malocclusion* was a factor. That said, it is dangerous and simplistic to consider any occlusion to be the *cause* of a multifactorial condition, such as TMD. In fact, to consider any occlusion to be a "malocclusion" is thought to be outdated by many dentists. In his paper in 2006, Gremillion [6] makes a useful distinction between the term "malocclusion" and his term of "maladaptive occlusion". In addition, it was argued in the BDJ in 2007 [7] that the term malocclusion [literally "bad bite"] is meaningless as it judges an occlusion by a set of rules suggested by Angle in 1899 and based upon the *Old Glory* dried skull.

The term "maladaptive occlusion" infers that the only valid judgement of an occlusion is by the patient's tissues reaction [or lack of] to it.

8.7 Comment

This patient has failed to adapt to the change in occlusion that seems to have occurred since a single tooth was removed.

Possible Aetiology: Another name for *a Premature Contact in Centric Relation* is a *Deflecting or Guidance Contact.* If the tooth that was removed was the Premature Contact in Centric Relation [CR], then it would have been the occlusal contact that *deflected* or *guided* the jaw movement to the patient's comfortable and familiar Habitual Bite [Centric Occlusion CO].

But if this hypothesis is accepted, then it is not difficult to imagine that the elimination of the Premature or Guidance Contact by extracting the tooth, in a *very small minority* of patients, could result in the loss of their comfortable and consistent bite.

8.8 Management

1. *Supported self-management*
    (a) The patient reported at the time of examination that there was an immediate benefit in being given an explanation of why this might be occurring.
    (b) Finding better coping strategies, including continuing to engage in social activities, taking time every day to complete an activity which brings joy and ensuring taking gentle exercise daily, was suggested to the patient to support general wellness.
2. *Muscle therapy*
    (a) Warm compresses at least three times a day, for a period of 6 weeks.
    (b) The patient was referred for physiotherapy.

3. *Splint therapy*: In this case, a single tooth extraction has led to change in occlusion to which patient has failed to acclimatise. In such cases, provision of a stabilisation splint early in the treatment phase alongside SSM would provide a more stable occlusal platform expected to be beneficial to reduce neuromuscular activity and support symptom reduction. In this case, an upper stabilisation splint alongside supported self-management strategies resulted in pain reduction and improved adaptation to "new bite" to the patient's delight.

9 Case History 9: Myofascial Pain Following Extensive Restorative Treatment

9.1 Patient's Aspiration

"I want to have a comfortable bite again, and to get rid of the pain in my face."

9.2 History of Presenting Complaint(s)

Site

"I have pain in my left cheek region and in front of my left ear, when I open my mouth."

Onset/Event

"All of this started after I had six crowns placed on my back teeth, 6 months ago."

Character of Pain and Severity

"The pain is continuous but varies in intensity. My teeth on the right hurt when they come into contact."

Associations/Timings

"I had a comfortable bite and no pain before I had crowns placed. I had had some of the teeth root filled by a specialist endodontist and some of the crowns replaced by another dentist who also made a hard splint. But neither the crowns nor the splint comfortable to close against. My pain has not improved."

Timings

"I didn't have any problems until I had those crowns placed."

Exacerbating/Relieving Factors

"It's just there, nothing makes it better or worse."

State of Mind or Mood

"This situation is exhausting and gets me down. I wish I had never had any treatment.

I am not the person I was before I had this treatment."

9.3 The Articulatory System Exam

Case 9 detailed articulatory exam is presented in Fig. 9.

Note the following key findings:

Temporomandibular Joint		Right	Left
Tender to palpation?	*Lateral pole*	no	no
	Causes Familiar PAIN	**N/A**	N/A
Noises? **No noises heard**	*Clicks*	Right Left Bilateral Soft Loud Consistent Intermittent [intermittent with .... Opening Closing Both Cycle: Early Mid Late Painful Painless Single Multiple	
	If patient has consistent clicks, do these clicks disappear when the patient opens from a protrusive mandibular position?		
	Crepitus	Right Left Bilateral Painful Painless	
Range of motion? (mm)	*Lateral*	R ← **8** | **9** → L	
MAXIMUM MOUTH OPENING: 39mm	*Vertical*	Str 39 ↓ Comfortable	

Muscle Tenderness ***MARK*** ★ ***IF Causes Familiar PAIN***

	Technique	Right	Left
Temporalis	Palpation	NO	No
Masseter	Palpation	Yes	Yes ★

Occlusion Record

Fig. 9 Case history 9, myofascial pain following extensive restorative treatment articulatory examination results

Skeletal	Class 2		
Angles	Class II div i		
Static occlusion	Does C.O occur in C.R? No		
	If not – premature contact in C.R? *Roughly:* *Consistent Left 1st Premolar region* *or* *Exactly* *Palatal cusp of upper right 1st premolar against lower right canine* *Direction of slide from C.R to C.O:* large slide: Horozontal and to LHS *Freedom in centric occlusion?* *Yes* Existing Hard Splint: not made in CR and provided a supra occlusion on the LHS		
Dynamic occlusion		**Right**	**Left**
	Non-working side interferences?	no	no
	Working side interferences?	-	-
	Crossover position: *Non-working side*	–	–
	Working side	-	-
	Canine guidance?	-	-
	Group function?	Yes	Yes

Excessive wear X *Evidence of tooth/restoration fracture* X

Cheek ridging yes *tongue scalloping* yes

Compression Test *Tongue Spatulae*	**Elicits Pre-Auricular Pain?**	
	Pain on RHS?	**Pain on LHS?**
on RHS	☐ No *myogenic*	☐ No *arthrogenic*
on LHS	☐ No *arthrogenic*	☐ yes *myogenic*

Fig. 9 (continued)

- No functional abnormalities detected with temporomandibular joint
- Strong evidence of muscle hypertonicity and discomfort
- Large slide from the premature contact in Centric Relation [Retruded Contact Position] to their (uncomfortable) Centric Occlusion [Maximum Intercuspation Position]
- Heavy posterior interferences

9.4 Further Investigations

Study models mounted on to articulator in Centric Relation; duplicated if any adjustment of the recently placed restorations is considered.

9.5 Diagnosis

- Broad group diagnosis: myogenous TMD (M-TMD)
- Specific TMD sub-classification: myofascial pain affecting bilateral masseters and temporalis

9.5.1 Important Features of this Case

- There is a suggestion of a *maladaptive* occlusion [6].
- Significant distress.
- History of multiple interventions without benefit.

9.6 Management

This patient had seen multiple practitioners without any benefit, and this had contributed to her distress. She needed a clear explanation for her symptoms, and a multidisciplinary approach to their management, and that she needed to be on that team and to persevere with suggested strategies to allow time for improvement. Expectations needed to be manages with regard to seeking an instant "fix" for these issues.

1. *Muscle Therapy*

   A significant element of this patient's discomfort is muscle based. It is, therefore, logical to provide treatment directly to the muscles. This has two benefits: firstly to make the patient more comfortable and secondly to improve function, which is an importance step towards restoring the patient to their former condition.

   Consequently:

   (i) Warm compresses
   (ii) Physiotherapy

2. *Splint therapy*

   The splint that had been made did not fulfil the criteria of a stabilisation splint, which did not mean that it was without merit as it gave the patient something different to clench against. Unfortunately, it had not provided any benefit. In order to progress the patient's care, adjustments were made to the splint to provide a balanced occlusion in Centric Relation that was free from posterior interferences. The patient found that this was significantly more comfortable, which gave them hope that it would be possible to return them to the comfort of their pre-restorative treatment state. Adjustments to the existing splint were done to provide a balanced occlusion in CR.

3. *Psychosocial: supported self management*

   The dental practitioner took time to listen to patient's issues, meet their expectations and explain pathogenesis in detail. This type of care was what was needed to empower the patient to engage in *supported* self-management at home. It may seem alien to some colleagues that we are encouraging this element of the management of TMD. In fact, some dentists may think psychosocial treatment to be out with their skill set, but this sort of engagement with patients is often the biggest marker of a successful prognosis.

   As a profession, it is not alien to provide comfort and reassurance to anxious patients; the authors are suggesting that this care can be extended to this group of patients.

9.7 Outcome of Management

Initial Treatment

(i) *Report from the dentist who had been supporting the patient's self-management*

"Overall there is a positive response to the strategies that we have discussed."

- "I was pleased to hear that she has felt able to reduce the use of the Stabilisation Splint. She is now still wearing it a night, but finds that 2 to 3 short sessions of about 30 min during the day is effective."
- I think that it is significant that she has felt able to go out and enjoy a meal with her family. Previously her discomfort and dysfunction had prevented her from engaging in this pleasurable activity.
- She reports that she is in "a happier place."
- "During our recent conversations, she seems to be much happier."

(ii) *Report from physiotherapist*

"There is a reduction in pain and tenderness and an improvement in muscle function."

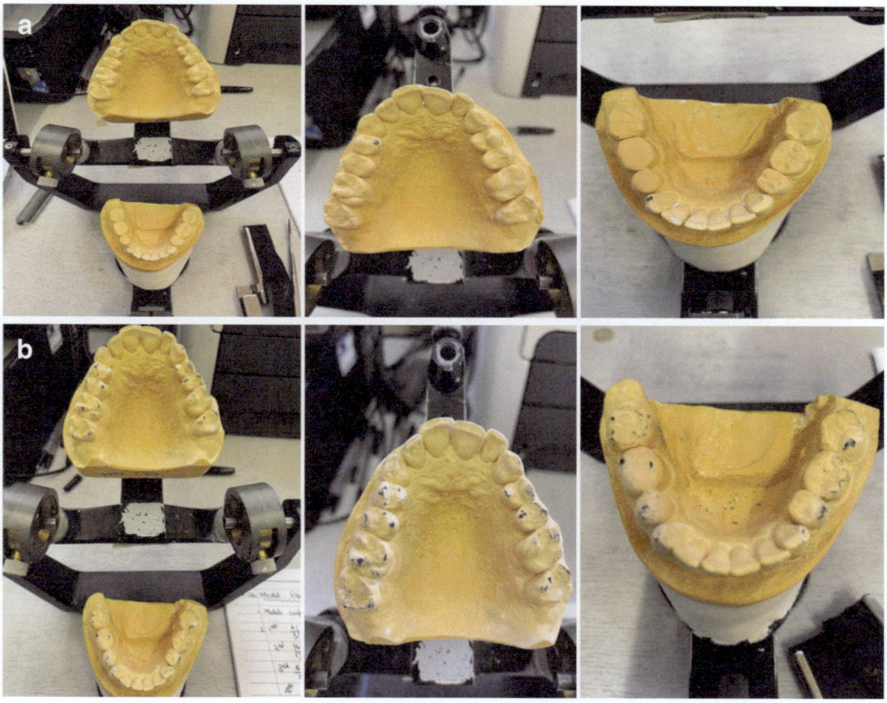

Fig. 10 Equilibration of models and then existing crown and teeth. (**a**) Premature contact in centric relation. (**b**) After equilibration of models demonstrating even ICP contacts around the arches

9.7.1 Specialist Referral

Alongside the conservative strategies for TMD and holistic wellness, the patient was referred for specialist assessment of the occlusal pattern. The specialist referral was made to a team adept at managing both pain and restorative dental needs to ensure best outcome. The specialist team mounted duplicate models to replicate the premature contact in Centric Relation and then carried out a "mock equilibration" on those models, shown in Fig. 10a, b [7]. This is a prerequisite to making any permanent changes to the teeth or crowns, no matter how minor.

Note: this is a complicated and precise exercise that requires specialist training and is rarely advocated. Occlusal adjustment should never be used as a first line of treatment for any TMD. It is a specialist treatment, and should not be undertaken by someone who has not undergone training, and even then only after the rehearsal on some accurately mounted models, on a semi-adjustable articulator. It is not "spot grinding".

References

1. Schiffman E, et al. Diagnostic Criteria for Temporomandibular Disorders (DC/TMD) for clinical and research applications: recommendations of the international RDC/TMD consortium network* and Orofacial Pain Special Interest Group†. J Oral Facial Pain Headache. 2014;28(1):6–27.
2. Eng R. Temporomandibular (TMD) online calculator and screening tool. 2024; Available from: https://www.rcseng.ac.uk/dental-faculties/fds/publications-guidelines/clinical-guidelines/tmd-guidelines-online-calculator/.
3. Beecroft E, Palmer J, Penlington C, Avery L, Aggarwal V, Chase M, Davies S, Gerber B, Jagger R, Harrison S, Horton M, Jones L, Kalantzis A, Lie S, McKenna G, McMillan R, Morton M, Murphy E, Renton T, Thayer T, Weden A, Durham J. Management of painful Temporomandibular disorder in adults NHS England Getting It Right First Time (GIRFT) and Royal College of Surgeons' Faculty of Dental Surgery. 2024; Available from: https://www.rcseng.ac.uk/dental-faculties/fds/publications-guidelines/clinical-guidelines/.
4. TMJA. Temporomandibular Joint Association: diet, nutrition and you. 2015; Available from: https://tmj.org/wp-content/uploads/2020/08/TMJ_nutrition_Guide.pdf.
5. Schiffman EL, et al. Longitudinal stability of common TMJ structural disorders. J Dent Res. 2017;96(3):270–6.
6. Gremillion HA. Relationship between TMD and occlusion. J Evid-Based Dent Pract. 2006;6:43–7.
7. Davies SJ. Malocclusion: a term in need of dropping or redefinition? Br Dent J. 2007;202:519–20.
8. Davies S. A guide to good occlusal practice. Springer; 2022. p. 97–102. https://doi.org/10.1007/9/978-3-030-79225-1. ISBN 978-3-030-79224-4.

The Role of the General Dental Practitioner in Temporomandibular Disorders

Stephen Davies

There are two reasons why it is important for the general dental practitioner (GDP) to consider temporomandibular disorders (TMD). The first concerns the care by the GDP of those patients who will present with the signs and symptoms of a TMD. The second is related to the articulatory system.

1 The Role of the GDP in the Diagnosis and Management of TMD

1.1 Do Dentists See Patients Who Are Suffering from a TMD?

The answer to this question is undoubtedly yes; all dentists will see patients who are suffering from one of the TMD subtypes. The prevalence of TMD in the general population combined with the proportion of the population who regularly attend a dentist makes it inevitable that every dentist will have seen a patient who has a TMD.

1.2 Do Dentists See [Diagnose] TMD in Their Patients?

This is not the same question, and it is less certain that TMD will be picked up during some dental examinations. There are probably two reasons for this.

Firstly, some of the symptoms of TMD might not naturally lead the patient to seek the opinion of their dentist especially given around a quarter first present complaining of a "headache" albeit situated in the temporal region. Another good example are patients who are suffering from pre-auricular pain who may assume it to be earache and therefore consult their doctor.

S. Davies (✉)
Division of Dentistry, University of Manchester, Manchester, UK
e-mail: stephen.j.davies@manchester.ac.uk

S. Davies et al. (eds.), *Temporomandibular Disorders in Primary Dental Care*, BDJ Clinician's Guides, https://doi.org/10.1007/978-3-032-01301-9_8

Secondly, unless the dentist is listening and looking for the symptoms and signs of a TMD and has used a reliable examination protocol, there is a danger that the patient's condition will go underdiagnosed. We all can only diagnose what we know, a fact that is termed *availability bias*. But in addition to the *missed diagnosis* that might be the result of a dentist not having the tools and knowledge to spot a TMD, there is another danger which is also unfortunate. That is a *mis*diagnosis.

Everyone who works in a secondary (specialist) care will have seen a patient who has been referred, often after sitting on a long waiting list, and sometimes after having received inappropriate and even irreversible treatment, and for whom a simple examination will indicate that *they do not* have a TMD. There can be a tendency to assume that a pain for which the GDP cannot find an obvious cause "must be a TMD"; whereas in reality, it may be anything from referred pulpal pain to a neuralgia. If a dentist cannot diagnose TMD, then they probably cannot determine that the patient *does not have TMD*, both a *missed diagnosis* and a *misdiagnosis* represent less than ideal care.

GDPs work in primary care, and as that nomenclature suggests, they are usually the first port of call for a patient. This has some benefits in terms of accessibility: it may be much easier for a patient to be seen by their GDP than in a secondary care facility, which means that the patient's condition is likely to be addressed *sooner*. This is a major advantage for TMD and will help improve prognosis if a diagnosis is given and management is started early. This improvement in prognosis is due to the fact that it is less likely that central sensitisation of the nociceptive system will have occurred. Once centrally sensitised changes have occurred, the successful management of the patient can become more complex. If the pain is of early onset, simple measures are more likely to be successful. Once the pain has become persistent, the patient may suffer from compounding factors that will make their recovery more difficult.

A GDP and a patient may also have a long-standing professional relationship, and because of that, the dentist is likely to know much more about the patient's condition and circumstances than will be gained from taking a history in a secondary care environment. This puts the primary care dentist in a better position than their secondary care counterpart to design an effective management plan and provide appropriate support. Because TMD are multi-factorial and their management nearly always requires a multi-disciplinary approach, it is important that we treat individual patients rather than adopting a *one-size-fits-all approach*. It is a huge advantage to have a knowledge of the patient's circumstances and aspirations. The effective care of an individual living with TMD is dependent not only upon the clinician's ability to make a diagnosis but their knowledge of the patient. This will mean that a management strategy can be devised that is appropriate for that individual patient.

The familiarity of the clinical environment and auxiliary staff may also be a comfort the patient (Fig. 1).

Even if a GDP does not feel able to diagnose and manage their patient's TMD, the familiarity that they have with their patient will enable them to make a referral

Fig. 1 Never treat a stranger

Different Patients with the Same Diagnosis
will get different Management Strategies,
because they a different people.
So, a knowledge of the patient as an
individual is an essential aid to designing
appropriate treatments

that contains much more information than the basic personal details and relevant medical history. For instance, it will provide a detailed account of:

- The signs and symptoms with relevant dates.
- Any exacerbating or relieving factors.
- Some information on the initiating, perpetuating or potentiating biopsychosocial factors.
- Previous treatments, with outcomes.
- Finally, it will be useful if some idea of the patient's expectations are outlined; this may vary from a simple reassurance to a hope that some other issue can be addressed.

The vast majority of TMD have a cyclic nature, meaning most cases will need continuing care. Review is, therefore, an important part of management. This ongoing care can relatively easily be built into a GDP's treatment plans. It is much more difficult to provide on a routine basis in secondary care.

Even if the patient is referred to a secondary care facility, then there is a professional obligation for the GDP to follow up their progress and influence aspects of their care they are comfortable managing. This will include promoting engagement with supported self-management strategies and providing longitudinal reassurance. General dental practices are usually staffed by a team of dental professionals. There is no reason why a trained dental nurse, hygienist and dental therapist should not take the responsibility of contacting the patient for regular reviews and organising a case review appointment with the GDP when indicated. The continuity of care that this might facilitate could be a valuable contribution to supported self-management.

2 The Articulatory System

As has already been stated, TMD can be paraphrased as a disorder, dysfunction or a discomfort within the articulatory system. This simplistic description is not instead of the diagnostic criteria that have been presented (Fig. 2).

If the reader accepts the existence of this system, there are several consequences:

Fig. 2 The three components of the articulatory system, together with their functions

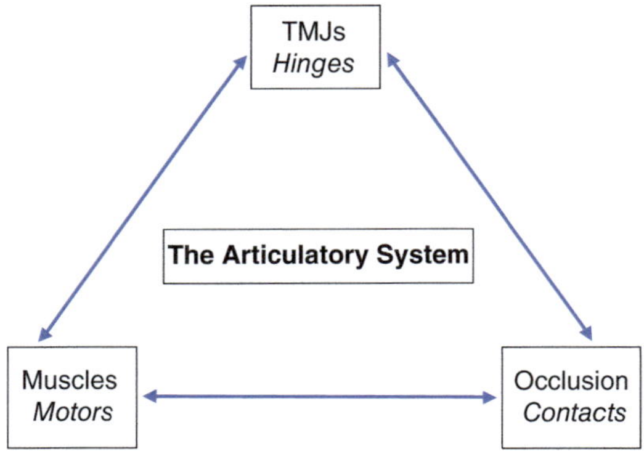

Fig. 3 The stomatognathic or masticatory system

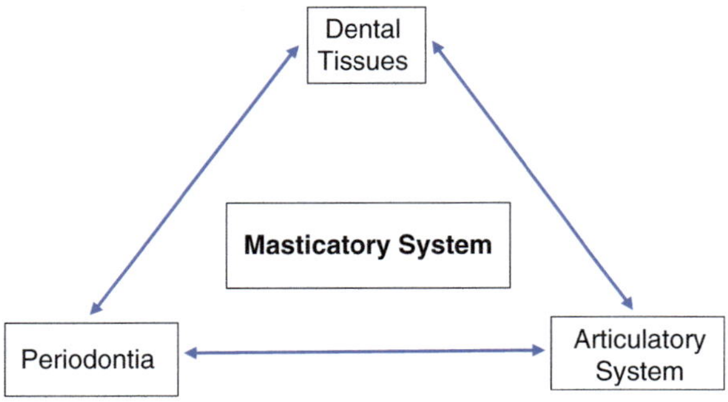

Firstly, just as the other two parts of the masticatory or stomatognathic system *need to be examined* as part of a comprehensive assessment of the patient, so the articulatory system warrants this attention (Fig. 3).

This examination is needed, maybe not as often, but it is recommended for:

- Every new patient
- Any patient suspected of suffering from a TMD
- Any patient for whom major changes in the occlusion is being planned

The articulatory system is a *system*. It is made up of interdependent and interrelated parts.

A change in one of the elements may change another element, but it is important to acknowledge that these changes are not necessarily always adverse.

As many dental treatments have the potential to change one part of the articulatory system, namely, the occlusion, it is essential for the dentist who is going to perform these treatments [orthodontics, major restorative treatments and prosthodontics, including implantology] to have examined the articulatory system before, during and after these treatments. This is not to say that a change in the occlusion may be associated with adverse reaction in the TMJs or muscles because the vast majority of patients will successfully adapt to any occlusal change, but cases do exist where an asymptomatic patient gives a history of a strong temporal relationship between some occlusally altering treatment and the onset of their symptoms. Examples of these unfortunate situations include:

- A patient who develops myalgia after fitted with a crown that is "high on the bite", and it does not "bed in" [or more likely the patient fails to adapt to the new occlusion].
- After the extraction of a single tooth, which with hindsight provided an important "centric stop", a patient may report that they cannot find a comfortable resting position to close their mouth. Some of these patients can go on to develop mandibular tremors and facial myalgia.
- If, during a course of treatment, an undiagnosed disc displacement with reduction [clicking] changes to a disc displacement without deduction with limited opening [closed lock], it may significantly impact on the dentist's ability to complete the treatment.
- If an extensive course of restorative treatment that cannot be provided to the conformative approach is not carefully planned and carried out to a predetermined occlusal prescription, then it is possible that the patient, in failing to adapt, will go on to develop chronic pain. As has already been discussed, this can result in significant emotional distress. From a restorative point of view, the management of this situation is very complex involving many stages of care, starting with an improvement in their TMD. It should be noted that if a patient fails to adapt to a new occlusion and its jaw relationship, returning to their pre-treatment occlusion/jaw relationship is not an option. That has been lost forever.
- Although the onset of a TMD is rare during orthodontic treatment, it is prudent to examine for a TMD before starting orthodontics.

It is important to realise that if a course of treatment exacerbates a pre-existing and undiagnosed TMD, a change in the occlusion may not be the cause. It may be the *process of* providing the treatment that was the major factor. If a dentist has a tendency to always blame the occlusion, and so start "adjusting the bite" often over multiple visits, they may perpetuate the difficulty that the patient is having to adjust to their new occlusion. It is much better to provide non-invasive and supportive treatment, possibly including splint therapy, as described in this book.

Discussion: Occlusion and TMD

This is dangerous ground to debate because the author is not saying that a change in the occlusion is the inevitable cause of a TMD. In fact, he has argued against this *mechanical perception* for many years, supporting the view that *Malocclusion* is a meaningless term [1] and supporting the use of the alternative term *Maladaptive* Occlusion [2, 3]. More recently, he has suggested that the restoration of a worn dentition [treatment involving a significant occlusal change] does not necessarily have to follow the complex but long-established rules of the re-organised approach, as long as the patient is monitored for any sign of an adverse reaction in the articulatory system [4]. But when a definite temporal relationship between a change in the occlusion and the onset of TMD signs and symptoms exists, it is hard not to make

Fig. 4 Is "Malocclusion" a useful term?

There is no such thing as an
intrinsically bad occlusion
[Malocclusion].

Only an intolerable number of times for that
individual patient
at that time in their life
to function or parafunction
on that occlusion
[Mal-Adaptive Occlusion]

Fig. 5 Can the patient improve their adaptation to their occlusion?

The aim of TMD treatment is to help
the patient into a higher level of
adaptive capability.
This is why psychosocial support is relevant
to their management

an unfavourable association or assume that the patient had an undetected pre-treatment TMD (Figs. 4 and 5).

The onset of symptoms of a TMD after a change in a patient's occlusion, either intended or unintended, is thankfully rare. But if it occurs, it can significantly adversely affect the patient's quality of life. To avoid this disaster for the patient's sake and from a medico-legal perspective, it is prudent to examine the articulatory system.

The good news is the examination protocol used to safeguard against these events is the same as is needed to detect TMD.

Because of this consideration, it is suggested that the examination protocols, diagnostic criteria and management strategies provided in this book are relevant to all dentists, not just those who have a special interest in TMD.

References

1. Davies SJ. Malocclusion–a term in need of dropping or redefinition? Br Dent J. 2007;202(9):519–20.
2. Gremillion HA. The relationship between occlusion and TMD: an evidence-based discussion. J Evid Based Dent Pract. 2006;6(1):43–7.
3. Davies SJ. Definition of ideal occlusion. In: A guide to good occlusal practice. Springer Nature; 2002.
4. Davies S, et al. Occlusion: is there a third way? A discussion paper. Br Dent J. 2021;231(3):160–2.

Correction to: Functional Anatomy and Pain Science

David Edwards, Joanna Matthan, James Allison, Emma Beecroft, Chris Penlington, and Justin Durham

Correction to:
Chapter 2 in: S. Davies et al. (eds.), *Temporomandibular Disorders in Primary Dental Care*, BDJ Clinician's Guides, https://doi.org/10.1007/978-3-032-01301-9_2

This book was inadvertently published with the incorrect spelling of author name and affiliation. This has now been amended throughout the book from Joanna Matten to Joanna Matthan along with affiliation "Newcastle University Medicine Malaysia (NUMed), Johor, Malaysia".

The updated version of this chapter can be found at
https://doi.org/10.1007/978-3-032-01301-9_2

S. Davies et al. (eds.), *Temporomandibular Disorders in Primary Dental Care*,
BDJ Clinician's Guides, https://doi.org/10.1007/978-3-032-01301-9_9

MIX
Papier aus verantwortungsvollen Quellen
Paper from responsible sources
FSC® C105338

If you have any concerns about our products,
you can contact us on
ProductSafety@springernature.com

In case Publisher is established outside the EU,
the EU authorized representative is:
Springer Nature Customer Service Center GmbH
Europaplatz 3, 69115 Heidelberg, Germany

Printed by Libri Plureos GmbH
in Hamburg, Germany